NATURAL
FIBROMYALGIA
CHOICES

FIND THE CAUSE AND
HEAL THE SYMPTOMS

Jane Oelke, ND, PhD

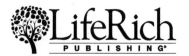
LifeRich
PUBLISHING®

LifeRich Publishing is a registered trademark of The Reader's Digest Association, Inc.

LifeRich Publishing books may be ordered through booksellers or by contacting:

LifeRich Publishing
1663 Liberty Drive
Bloomington, IN 47403
www.liferichpublishing.com
1 (888) 238-8637

ISBN: 978-1-4897-2189-1 (sc)
ISBN: 978-1-4897-2187-7 (hc)
ISBN: 978-1-4897-2188-4 (e)

Library of Congress Control Number: 2019903377

Print information available on the last page.

LifeRich Publishing rev. date: 03/26/2019

Acknowledgments

There are many supportive people I want to acknowledge in helping me complete this book. Thanks to the 50 research participants in the bio-chemical research project almost 20 years ago. Some of them are now long-term clients, and many of them are better now than they were in 1999. All of my clients' dedication to noticing their health and providing feedback on what helps them is appreciated. The suggestions I commonly make for them generated the many recommendations in this book.

I also want to acknowledge the ongoing support of Johannes Fisslinger and the Specialists at Lifestyle Prescriptions® University. They continue to teach me how to find the real cause of symptoms, and ways to use detailed techniques to help clients balance mental and emotional fitness. I observed these concepts for many years. The organized way the information is taught now makes it clear and useful for practitioners and clients. Their growing list of Lifestyle Prescriptions® Health Coaches help many people around the world revitalize their health.

Contents

What Is Fibromyalgia?

Fibromyalgia is a chronic pain syndrome that affects many people. I want to give hope to people with fibromyalgia that there are effective ways to get rid of this pain. Back in 2001, I did a study to measure metabolic imbalances in people with fibromyalgia pain. Since then many new studies and even commercials now agree with my findings that fibromyalgia is caused by nervous system stress that makes muscles cry out in pain. Your muscles and nerves are telling you constantly, "Pay attention to me!" Fibromyalgia is one of the auto-immune syndromes that continue to affect more and more people. Many of the following recommendations for fibromyalgia will also help most other auto-immune conditions like rheumatoid arthritis, systemic lupus erythematosus, inflammatory bowel disease, and multiple sclerosis.

Doctors used to tell people with fibromyalgia pain that their pain was "all in their head," but that has been disproven. Most medications for fibromyalgia used to be anti-depressants, but that has changed also. Now there are new medications, but the side-effects can be worse than the pain. I coach many clients with fibromyalgia, and here I will share practical ideas to reduce chronic pain by creating the cellular energy you need. I see many people relieved of their chronic pain and get improved energy with a variety of natural choices. You will use quizzes and procedures to evaluate how you are improving using these ideas.

We are going to explore six relating elements to help you figure out the root cause of your fibromyalgia pain. The six elements are Organ Tissue, Stress Triggers, Emotions, Beliefs, Social and Lifestyle. Each of these elements has overlapping relationships that will show you how and why our brain creates pain responses. Your body and mind are connected and exchange information continuously. Psychological and social factors trigger your central nervous system causing chronic pain after injuries or stressful events do not resolve adequately. The way you think and respond to stress influences how you experience life physically, emotionally and energetically.

Pain is a signal that the body is lacking energy in the muscles and to heal they need more voltage or energy in the cells. This lack of power in your cells affects your nervous system and muscle response. Low energy is what causes the most common fibromyalgia symptoms:

- Stiffness from congestion in the tissues
- Chronic pain
- Hypersensitivity
- Extreme fatigue
- Sleep disturbances
- Brain fog
- Anxiety/depression

To relieve these symptoms, we need to get more energy in the tissues by improving metabolism. Then our nervous system and connective tissues will have better circulation and much less pain. By recognizing what areas to improve specifically, you will be able to know the cause and what to do to feel better quickly.

Soon, you will understand how to identify fibromyalgia and fibromyalgia-related symptoms. You will see how stress affects metabolism, and how to measure the effects of this stress. If you don't support your metabolism, the effects of excess stress will continue to grow, creating more symptoms in various parts of your body.

You will learn how daily nutritional choices can support your body to rebuild tissue. Poor food choices and excess acids in your system cause weakness in your tissues. You will begin to notice the effects of acid and alkaline balance in your tissues and know how to do saliva and urine testing to see the direction of your health. You will discover the source of free radical activity that essentially causes our body to "rust," or age more quickly.

Even though everyone is affected by stress, the health of your metabolism will determine your susceptibility to specific disorders. You will discover common symptoms that relate to metabolism imbalances and connect them to the known benefits of homeopathic remedies, nutritional supplements, and natural health techniques. And you will learn how to recognize which techniques and remedies will benefit you the most. All of the information is designed to help people with fibromyalgia; yet, also assists those who want to be healthy and prevent chronic pain or auto-immune disease.

The Philosophy of Natural Healing

Natural health techniques are designed to work with the intelligence our body has to stay healthy. This inner wisdom of the body directs and controls every function of every cell. Symptoms are warning signals from this innate intelligence that we are compromising our state of health. Symptoms are indicators that we have stress in a specific part of our body, and we are now in the process of correcting the problem.

Symptoms show up during the healing process. For example, when we have a "cold," a runny nose is a cleansing reaction to a toxic build-up that has occurred. If we suppress these cold symptoms, the body does not have a chance to heal fully, causing a recurrence, a deeper imbalance, or disease process later on. Asthma and bronchitis are two of the deeper imbalances that can occur when we suppress cold symptoms repeatedly.

Many doctors that use natural healing techniques do not diagnosis a disease name. Patients do not get better by identifying the disease name. They may lose hope when a diagnosis is made for a supposedly incurable disease. By looking at the specific individual symptoms, naturopathic doctors recognize imbalances and use coaching, remedies, and hands-on techniques to stimulate the innate natural healing ability to bring the body back towards health. Using natural health techniques is more than just prevention of disease; it is supporting and maintaining a consistent state of health.

We produce symptoms as a warning signal that we have done something to disturb the natural balance. If the body has the intelligence to generate a disease profile; by removing the cause, it is also capable of reversing the process and creating health. Our body always attempts to maintain health and compensates as best it can under the circumstances. For many of us, this compensation causes symptoms that relate to disease profiles. By removing the disturbance, whether it is physical or emotional, the cells in the body will change their function and return to health. Usually, the longer the body is in the stress phase, the longer it will take to reverse the symptoms.

Do you realize that we create a new stomach lining every 3 to 4 days, a new skin layer every four weeks, and a new liver every five months? So, why don't we recreate a healthy liver, or why does our skin continue to have eczema? It is because energy blockages in our cells cause our body to forget how it should function and we stay with what we know as "normal" now. Our organ tissues recreate the same pattern of illness because that is what it remembers from our habits. You will learn how to help your tissues get back to ideal balance by retraining your cells to react correctly, thereby reversing illness profiles.

Homeopathic philosophy believes that a person is not sick because he has an illness, but that he has an illness because he is sick. The illness is the symptom profile showing up, and the sickness is the metabolic imbalance causing the symptoms. It is imperative to find the cause of the symptoms to truly promote healing. Homeopathic remedies are energetic remedies that can help sustain optimal health. Specialized homeopathic combination remedies remind your body how to function properly after it has lost its memory on what to do.

Specific remedies promote healthy new tissue regeneration, and you will learn how to use these remedies to reduce pain.

Our healing ability depends on the vitality of the body. By definition, the vitality refers to the overall energy level of the body, how well blood circulates nutrients into the cells, and how free the tissues are from toxins. The higher the vitality, the more energy the cells will have to release the toxins and remove them from the body. The skin and mucous membranes will be the most common ways toxins will exit when the vitality is high. When the vitality lowers, due to an increase in stress or toxic buildup, the body does not have the energy to release toxins and will store them in the tissues causing congestion and fibromyalgia pain.

Your tissues always use your available energy to keep your metabolism in the best condition possible. Some fibromyalgia patients find this hard to accept as true. It is difficult for them to believe the pain associated with fibromyalgia is a warning sign telling them to do something different from what they are doing now. So it is essential to figure out what you need to change, in order to make a difference in your health.

Better Health through Awareness

My Natural Choices business motto is "Better Health through Awareness." I feel it is essential to gain knowledge that can help me make better decisions on what is best for my body. Not all of us will get fibromyalgia pain with a compromised nervous system. But for those that do, it is vital to know what is causing the symptoms. While my specialty is homeopathy, I also do biochemical nutritional testing. My previous background as a research engineer has provided me with extensive interest in scientifically demonstrating proven ways to help people.

I did a biochemical research project back in 1999 to measure and compare the relationship of symptoms found in fibromyalgia clients to metabolic imbalances. This research project was performed using 50 volunteers who had been diagnosed with fibromyalgia and compared their results to 50 other clients who did not have fibromyalgia. By comparing the fibromyalgia client's readings with the control group's results, I was able to see what type of metabolic imbalances cause fibromyalgia pain.

The idea for the research project came from a seminar I taught to nurses called Natural Choices for Fibromyalgia. Much of the information presented in the seminar correlated metabolic imbalances to fibromyalgia symptoms. When working individually with clients having fibromyalgia, most of the relief came when the client was able to improve their metabolism. Therefore, this research project was designed to find specific correlations between biochemical test results and fibromyalgia symptoms.

To understand the variety of differences between each person diagnosed with fibromyalgia, each participant in the research project filled out a questionnaire. Information requested in this questionnaire included their age, when and how fibromyalgia began, the number of tender points that tested positive, and the main locations of pain. The purpose of the questionnaire was to make sure that all of the participants understood how fibromyalgia is diagnosed and to confirm that they had the symptoms related to the syndrome.

Fibromyalgia affects mainly women most often when they are in their forties and fifties. Of the 50 participants who were part of the fibromyalgia group, 4 were men, and 46 were women. The average age for the participants was 49.7 years old. The ages of the participants ranged between 19 and 85 years old. As people age, they are more prone to fibromyalgia symptoms. You will understand why as we explore the various causes of fibromyalgia.

We will focus on the effects of how stress, emotions, beliefs, and lifestyle affect our organs and social environment. Acidity, adrenal stress, mineral levels, and oxidative stress are metabolic factors relating to pain responses. We will see how diet and nutritional supplementation can be used effectively to reduce pain. We will also look at how homeopathic remedies reduce stress levels, improve metabolic function, and drain toxins. I believe both types of support are needed, especially in the initial stages of reversing symptoms. Homeopathic remedies often reduce pain more quickly while nutritional support physically nourishes the muscles and nervous system. Together they help maintain healthy metabolic balances.

Healing occurs in layers and phases. Often during a first consultation, we focus on reducing overall stress, so the client is ready for more in-depth healing responses. Doing too many changes or too many remedies or supplements at first can overwhelm the body and mind. Begin by peeling layers of stress away, similar to peeling an onion. Often we don't know the deeper levels of healing needed until we uncover the top layers. As we get closer to the core symptom, we gain a more profound long-term healing response. When we have chronic disease patterns, we go through phases of healing that we have to honor and understand as part of our innate healing intelligence.

The Five Phases of Self-Healing

Why do we get symptoms of pain or sickness? Could there be a process that the body follows in creating a healing response? Have you ever been "sick" after a stressful event? Or do you get "sick" on vacation? Our body's innate intelligence follows a cycle to react to daily stressful events we experience so that we can stay healthy.

It is essential to understand how our nervous system works, so we can be aware of why we are having specific reactions. The autonomic nervous system is part of the peripheral nervous system that regulates metabolic processes that take place without conscious effort. The autonomic system is responsible for controlling involuntary body functions such as heartbeat, blood flow, breathing, and digestion, areas where we usually do not pay attention.

The autonomic nervous system keeps our body's internal environment in balance, known as homeostasis. The autonomic nervous system controls our body temperature, blood sugar, mineral balance, body weight, oxygen levels, and heart rate. The autonomic nervous system also plays a significant role in how we experience emotions. When we get emotionally excited, we will notice that our heart rate increases, our mouth may become dry, and our stomach may feel queasy.

The autonomic nervous system operates by receiving information from the outside environment and other parts of the body. The autonomic nervous system has two components that work in contrasting ways. The sympathetic nervous system will usually stimulate a response, and the parasympathetic nervous system will inhibit it. Generally, the sympathetic system is a quick response system that mobilizes the body for action, where the parasympathetic system is believed to act more slowly to dampen responses, returning your body to its normal, resting state.

The sympathetic nervous system prepares the body for stressful emergencies that cause a fight/flight/freeze response. Typical reactions are increases in heart rate and the force of heart contractions, along with dilating the airways to make breathing easier. Stored energy from the liver is released, and muscle strength increases. The sympathetic division also causes sweaty palms, pupils to dilate, and hair to stand on end. It slows other body processes that can wait until the emergency is over, like digestion. When the sympathetic nervous system is more active, it is making sure we have the energy to respond. When it is overactive, you will notice more tension, sleeplessness, cold extremities, high blood pressure, and obsessive thinking.

When we experience a stress event, the sympathetic nervous system starts to react. We often try to avoid the stress by ignoring it, known as a flight response. Or we fight the stress by taking action quickly to defend ourselves. Or we can freeze, or not respond to the stress. Like an opossum that plays dead when attacked, we can hold on to the stress in our tissues to handle it later. Emotional stress can get trapped in our tissues with a freeze response.

We do our best to solve the stress by stimulating metabolic factors. Generally, during this sympathetic state, you don't feel any pain because your body is operating at a heightened emergency level. There are underlying changes in organ tissues to support you through this process. We can't stay in this stressed state forever, so the body learns how to react so that when this stress happens again, we have a solution. Once there is a solution, the body begins the regeneration cycle where restoration and normalization of the organ tissue occurs. Then we switch to activating the parasympathetic nervous system.

The parasympathetic nervous system helps maintain normal body functions and conserves our physical resources. It helps to balance the reactions of the sympathetic nervous system to replace and recover from stressful events. It also controls the bladder, slows heart rate, and constricts pupils in the eye. The parasympathetic state stimulates digestion, so that nutrient absorption happens. It also reduces blood pressure.

In the parasympathetic state, we go into regeneration and normalization activities in organ tissues. In the parasympathetic state, we feel more tired, will have more pain responses, and feel warmer and inflamed. In certain circumstances, we may never solve the stressful event, and we stay in the stress phase while our body continues to locate a regeneration solution, showing as a chronic disease pattern.

We experience these different systems regularly. For example, our body is mostly in a sympathetic state during the day, and then at night we enter the parasympathetic state. After a shocking and stressful event, however, the body stays in the sympathetic state until a solution occurs for the issue. The body then goes into the parasympathetic state. At night, if we've experienced a shock earlier in the day and are in the sympathetic state, we may find that we can't sleep well; we'll toss and turn and sleep lightly. Often, the night before an important job interview we will be in a stressful state and have trouble sleeping. A sleepless night is not unusual in this situation. Once the job interview is over, and the stress resolves, you will want to rest for a while to regenerate.

The five phases of self-healing are managed first by the sympathetic nervous system, and then by the parasympathetic nervous system. Think about it this way; every morning we wake up and function during the day and then sleep at night. If we are awake too long, our body will be in a constant stress state. When we don't get enough sleep, then we don't give our body time to regenerate, and eventually, we will get symptoms. So each day we go through a stress and regeneration cycle.

Another example of the self-healing cycle is progressive weight training with gradual increases in pounds used to activate muscle fibers. When we do weight training regularly, we stress our muscles on purpose with excess weight, and our muscles have to relax, or they will create lactic acid and excess pain. If we constantly overly stress our muscles, they will eventually tear and not heal well.

Five Phases of Self-Healing

1. **Stress Trigger** - Stress triggers happen when we experience an initial traumatic event that completely catches us unprepared. During this time the brain records everything we see, hear, feel, taste, smell, and certain words are recognized and stored. Stressful events affect our thinking, trap emotions in specific tissues, and change how we react socially to our environment.

Another type of stress trigger is a conditioned reflex. A conditioned reflex occurs when we often re-visit a previous trauma or a significant emotional event, either internally or by telling others about it. By visually repeating the memory, or frequently telling the story about our traumatic event, we create a familiar pattern in the limbic system of our brain. Comparable to crafting a new habit, we create automatic responses through visual, auditory, or sensory experiences that remind us of our signature event. The limbic system in our brain has an organ called the amygdala. The amygdala helps you remember emotional events, and stores post-traumatic reflex stress events. Chronic pain cycle responses come from conditioned reflexes.

2. **Stress Phase** - A stress phase occurs when the sympathetic nervous system is active. We will tend to be cold, crave sugar to compensate for adrenal stress, or take medications or drink alcohol to avoid feeling this stress. Often compulsive thoughts begin in this phase creating belief patterns that hold us back from finding a solution. Because blood is directed away from the digestive system to the vital organs, we lose our appetite; have nausea, and acid reflux. Extra sugar goes into the cells and adrenalin increases so we can react faster. Insomnia is often seen in this phase, too.

Depending on the organ tissue function in our body, there will be a growth of fungi, bacteria, or a virus that will generate but remain dormant until the regeneration phase. Depending on how much the organ tissue is affected in the stress phase; microbes will be created in direct proportion to fix the tissues damaged during the stress phase.

We have ten times more microbes in our body than actual organ tissues. Each of these microbes has a function to help repair or rebuild tissues after a stress response. Viruses are produced during this time depending on the amount of cell reduction. When we don't have the required fungi, bacteria, or viruses in our system, then the body will get them from our outside environment, or they won't be produced, and other metabolic reactions will occur.

Typical symptoms of the Stress Phase depend on the type of organ tissues affected. Often there is constipation, weakness in muscles, excessive energy, dryness of the skin, a decrease in senses, and thickening of the dermis layer of the skin.

3. **Regeneration Trigger** - A regeneration trigger event can be conscious or unconscious. At this moment, the stress trigger is

resolved either with or without our awareness. The trauma ends, or a new solution is found. A solution can even happen during sleep as an unconscious fix. You wake up with a cold, having gone to bed feeling fine. At this point, the regeneration symptoms start to appear, and we will begin to experience the feelings of repairing the tissues affected during the stress phase.

4. **Regeneration Phase** - This restoration phase starts just after a solution to the stress is found. Now the parasympathetic nervous system is activated, and the body goes into repairing the damage made during the stress phase. This phase often creates "sick" symptoms depending on organ tissue affected. Some of the common symptoms are pain, congestion, edema, sensitivity to touch, and fatigue. While there was a reduction in cell thickness during the stress stage to allow more blood to flow, now to get back to homeostasis it has to go back to a normal thickness. When muscles repair, the most common symptoms are swelling and then stiffness and pain.

Our body's energy switches from fight/flight/freeze responses to repairing itself in this Regeneration Phase. During this restoration process, we get hot, sweaty, tired, feel ill, and ache all over. We want only to rest, and we should. There is an increase in secretions because of mucous membranes repair. For many people, this helps to explain recurring colds, coughs, and bronchitis.

Bacteria, viruses, and fungi produced during the Stress Phase support the actions of the Regeneration Phase depending on the type of tissue affected. In some organ tissues there is an increase in cell growth during the Stress Phase, so during the repair stage, the extra cells are eaten away by bacteria or fungi to return to homeostasis. If there are not enough good bacteria to remove the excess cells, then cysts form to encapsulate the organ tissue to be dealt with later.

Often right in the middle of the regeneration phase, a healing peak occurs. A healing peak is a short sympathetic nervous system response that occurs during the middle of the regeneration phase. It is a test for the mind and body that can cause an intense reaction like muscle twitching or spasms, or excessive urination when the body is getting rid of edema.

After the healing peak, we go into the second half of the regeneration phase where our body normalizes cell metabolism towards homeostasis. The parasympathetic nervous system is replenishing our energy reserves. We will feel more normal, but we may be hungrier as we want to rebuild our ability to deal with the stress if it occurs again. In the second part of the regeneration cycle, your muscle tissue increases, your bones become stronger, and you may develop scars. At this point, we will often notice drainage of toxins showing up as excess mucus and coughing.

5. **Health** – This is when we feel better, have a balanced metabolism, sleep well, and have good energy again.

These 5 phases of the self-healing process can be short, lasting only a few minutes, or can go on for days. Or they can be a long chronic process where the sympathetic stress trigger creates a conditioned reflex that is activated repeatedly through emotions, beliefs, lifestyle, or social interactions.

A chronic process begins when we stay in a sympathetic nervous state due to an unresolved stress event or a conditioned reflex. If a profoundly intense stressful experience continues for a long time, it may cause fatigue in organ tissues, high blood pressure, adrenal fatigue, or chronic pain. In chronic developments, the stress/regeneration cycle repeats again and again. You can see a diagram of these 5 Phases of Self-Healing on the cover of this book inside the circle of the 6 Root Causes of Symptoms.

6 Root Causes of Symptoms

In the following sections, we will look into causes and solutions for fibromyalgia. These are the topics we will cover to help heal from fibromyalgia. (Fisslinger, 2018)

Organ Tissue – See how specific organ tissues affect pain and how fibromyalgia is currently identified. We look at the function of the muscles, connective tissues, nerves, adrenals, and thyroid.

Stress Triggers – See how to recognize stress and trauma, and how it affects organ healing phases. Discover how specific stress conflicts relate to organ tissues.

Emotions – Emotions are energy in motion. Learn how trapped emotions affect organ tissue and how to identify and balance emotions.

Beliefs / Values – Understand how limiting beliefs affect our health, and how incongruent values affect stress responses.

Social – Realize how our relationships affect our health. Also learn how environmental toxins and microbial imbalance create symptoms, and find out how to release toxins effectively.

Lifestyle – Daily habits affect our health. Realize how to create better energy, sound sleep, and the effect of dietary choices. Also understand how acidity, oxidative stress, and absorption of nutrients affect health and learn recommendations for improvement.

The next sections will include solutions to reverse the various causes of pain. Improving your awareness of the cause of your pain will help you justify making better nutritional choices and stress reduction activities. Then in the final action plan section, you will be able to put together your program to fit your needs after learning therapies you can do.

Fibromyalgia Pain Quizzes

Before we go into the 6 Root Causes of Symptoms, I want to help you understand how your brain may be creating pain now. Here are six quizzes to help you evaluate where you need the most support to get free from fibromyalgia pain. There is an online version at my website – www.NaturalChoicesForYou.com. Using the results from the quizzes, you will be able to focus on the areas that are most important for you. Complete the quizzes here now, so you can go back in the future to monitor your progress:

Directions: Write   0 - not a symptom for you
                        1 - less than once a month
                        2 - weekly, or more than four times per month
                        3 - daily, or more than three times per week

Total the amount at the end of each quiz to see where you need to apply habit changes. You can find the section related to each of these categories in the following chapters.

Energy Metabolism Quiz

_____ Too tired to do what I want to do
_____ Wake up unrefreshed
_____ Have chronic muscle aches or weakness
_____ Have chronic infections

_____ Feel irritable and moody
_____ Tired after exercise
_____ Trouble falling asleep or staying asleep
_____ Feel depressed often
_____ Poor memory and concentration
_____ Exposed daily to pesticides, household chemicals, or radiation
_____ **Total**

Stress and Adrenal Fatigue Quiz

_____ Panic attacks
_____ Feel tired and wired
_____ Get fatigued easily
_____ Reccurring headaches
_____ Crave sugar
_____ Crave salt
_____ Get dizzy when rising
_____ Tired even after sleeping well
_____ Have trouble falling asleep or staying asleep all night
_____ Cannot concentrate
_____ **Total**

Thyroid Quiz

_____ Have cold hands or feet
_____ Have thin hair or lose many hairs daily
_____ Frequently constipated
_____ Loss of eyebrow hair on outside edges
_____ Have dry skin
_____ Weak sex drive
_____ Weak memory and concentration
_____ Swollen hands or feet
_____ Tend to be depressed
_____ **Total**

Digestion Quiz

_____ Have heartburn or take anti-acids daily
_____ Have fullness or bloating after eating
_____ Tired after eating
_____ Less than one bowel movement per day
_____ Have food reactions
_____ Crave sweets and bread
_____ Have undigested food in my stool
_____ Have recurring yeast infections
_____ Stools have a strong odor
_____ **Total**

Oxidative Stress Quiz

_____ Exposed to environmental chemicals daily at home or work
_____ Sensitive to fragrances, smoke, and chemical odors
_____ Have colds or sinus infections more than once per year
_____ Eat more than two servings of processed (boxed, microwave) meals daily
_____ Eat sugary treats or white flour products more than twice per week.
_____ Eat less than five servings of fruit and vegetables per day
_____ Exercise less than 30 minutes 3 times per week
_____ Drink more than three alcoholic drinks per week
_____ Smoke cigarettes or are exposed to cigarette smoke daily
_____ **Total**

Toxic Quiz

_____ Less than one bowel movement per day
_____ Drink tap water or soft drinks instead of filtered water
_____ Sensitive to caffeine (effects stay in the system for a long time)
_____ Sensitive to perfumes and other smells

_____ React to MSG and other preservatives
_____ Treat my home for insects more than once per year
_____ Have more than two mercury fillings in my mouth
_____ Sweat less than three times per week
_____ Have headaches often
_____ Exposed to chemicals at work or home daily
_____ **Total**

What are the top 3 areas for you to focus on in the following chapters?

1. _____

2. _____

3. _____

Organ Tissue

How Do I Know If I Have Fibromyalgia?

By definition, fibromyalgia is a chronic disorder characterized by widespread muscle, ligament, and tendon pain, with stiffness and tenderness on touch, lasting longer than three months, usually accompanied by fatigue, anxiety, and depression. In January of 1993, the World Health Organization officially declared fibromyalgia syndrome as the most common cause of widespread chronic muscle pain. The World Health Organization states that people with fibromyalgia syndrome might also experience other symptoms such as headaches, insomnia, cold sensitivity, restless leg syndrome, morning stiffness, and irritable bowel syndrome.

Fibromyalgia is called a syndrome, not a disease, since it represents a group of common nonspecific disorders characterized by pain, tenderness, and stiffness in muscles, ligaments, tendons, and adjacent connective tissues. Muscles, ligaments, tendons, and connective tissues are considered "fibrous" tissues. "Myalgia" is a medical term that indicates pain in the muscles, while "myositis" indicates inflammation of the muscle tissues. Fibromyalgia used to be called fibromyositis. (Wolf, 1986). However, inflammation is not the cause of fibromyalgia pain. Therefore, the term "fibromyalgia" is used to diagnose pain found in the fibrous tissues, muscles, ligaments, tendons, and connective tissues from non-specific causes. (NFA) Any of the fibrous tissues in the body may be involved, but the most common sites include widespread pain in the head, neck, shoulders, low back, hips, thighs, and knees.

In 2001, the American College of Rheumatology said that fibromyalgia affected 3 to 6 million Americans. (Wolfe, 1990) According to 2010 estimates by the National Fibromyalgia Association, fibromyalgia has grown to affect approximately 10 million people in the United States. (Jones, 2014) The majority are women between the ages of 25 and 60 years old, with females outnumbering males by 6:1. (Campbell, 1983; 26) There are possible reasons for this syndrome affecting women, which we will discuss in the emotions and stress sections.

Many fibromyalgia patients hold their stress internally, and may or may not appear tense, depressed, or anxious. The symptoms are often intensified by physical or mental stress, mental overactivity, sleep disorders, physical or emotional trauma, depression, exposure to dampness, heat, or cold, and occasionally by another disease process. (Wolfe, 1990) A viral or other systemic infection may bring on the syndrome in someone who is susceptible due to a weakened immune system. Patients often trace the onset of symptoms to an acute event or viral-like illness. Fibromyalgia may also be a complication of hypothyroidism or diabetes. Men are more likely to develop localized fibromyalgia in association with a particular occupational or recreational strain, or as a complication of sleep apnea. (Wilke, 1996L 100(1)) We will look at all of these physical and emotional factors in the following chapters.

Pain is the most common symptom of fibromyalgia. Fatigue is the second most common symptom associated with fibromyalgia. This fatigue is both physical and mental. Physically, the muscles feel tired or weak due to low energy reserves. Any regular activity, like shopping, walking upstairs and routine household responsibilities can tire the body quickly. Mental fatigue includes concentration problems, confused thoughts, and memory weakness. People with fibromyalgia tend to become more forgetful and absentminded than the average person. Forgetfullness happens because the brain is so busy being bombarded by pain signals, it has very little energy left to perform cognitive thinking. Headaches are also frequent and can feel like tension or migraine headaches. Tension headaches are the result of muscle contractions that usually begin in the neck, and travel up into the head area. Sleep disturbances are also common symptoms. Trouble falling asleep, or frequently waking throughout the night, does not allow the body the precious time required to restore itself.

Numbness and tingling, especially in the arms and legs, are common neurological disorders associated with fibromyalgia. Tingling may affect the hands and feet with feelings similar to carpal tunnel syndrome, or the sensation as if they were asleep. Tingling can affect the ability to use the hands or walk normally. Dizziness is another neurological disorder associated with fibromyalgia. Light-headedness and balance problems are the cause for lack of coordination. Weakness is another neurological complaint. This loss of strength and stamina creates deeper feelings of fatigue. Leg cramps in the calves, or restlessness in the legs when in bed at night, are also commonly associated symptoms of fibromyalgia.

Eighteen Tender Points

Everyone feels pain at some time in his or her life. Pain is a typical response of our nervous system to danger in our environment. The normal transmission of pain begins at specialized nerve endings in the skin, muscles, bones and other tissues. When heat from a hot stove touches our skin, the specialized nerve endings on our hands respond by releasing neurotransmitters that create tiny electrical currents through the spinal cord and into our brain. We do not realize the sense of pain until it reaches our brain, which happens in just milliseconds. This realization of pain also sends back a signal to the motor nerves in our hands to pull away from the hot stove.

The pain of fibromyalgia is different than this reactive pain response. Even though each person perceives pain differently, and can accommodate certain levels of pain, the pain of fibromyalgia creates a persistent pain that cannot be ignored. It is opposite of the normal accommodation we usually have for pain. For example, when we get into a hot tub, it is very hot at first, then when our body gets used to the heat, it accommodates to the heat. However, in fibromyalgia, the nervous system is not able to adapt to painful responses. When the pain becomes continuous, and it is difficult to find anything to relieve the pain, then it is time to check the correlation of the persistent symptoms to those of fibromyalgia syndrome.

Fibromyalgia is difficult to diagnose because many of the symptoms mimic those of other disorders. Muscle soreness in one spot, like the neck or lower back, cannot be diagnosed as fibromyalgia. There are different types of pain found in fibromyalgia. Some people experience aching pain, others feel sharp, stabbing pain sensations throughout their body. Other people feel burning pain, and some people experience a combination of all these types of pain.

In 2010, the American College of Rheumatology eliminated the need to include a tender point exam to diagnose fibromyalgia. Now more symptoms such as chronic fatigue, brain fog, and poor sleep are included as part of fibromyalgia syndrome. Now, to be classified with fibromyalgia, you have moderate pain with higher levels of other symptoms, or have moderate levels of other symptoms with higher all over pain, for at least three months, with no other cause to justify the pain.

Before 2010, the diagnosis for fibromyalgia included pressing on 18 tender, painful spots. When 11 or more of these points were tender, then it confirmed a fibromyalgia diagnosis. (Wolfe, 1990) These points are explained below along with a diagram.

1. On the back of the head at the lower edge of the skull, on both sides of the spine.
2. On both sides of the neck along the crease between the head and neck.
3. Mid-point on top of the shoulder in the muscle along the back edge of the shoulder called the trapezius.
4. On both sides of the spine, in the middle of the upper back just above the scapula or shoulder bone.
5. On the front, between the first and second rib in the upper chest area on both sides of the sternum.
6. On the inner side of the lower arm, about two inches down from the fold in the elbow.
7. On the lower back, near the dimpled area of the backside.
8. Along the side of the body in the middle hip area.
9. The inner side toward the back of the knee.

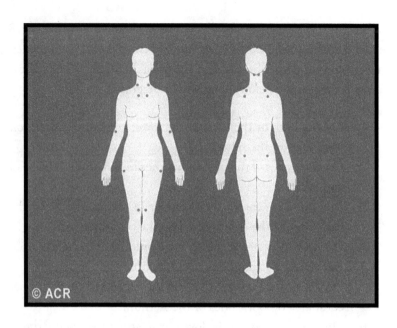

© ACR

Fibromyalgia Tender Points (ACR, 2010)

These points are pressed lightly and then pushed more strongly with a thumb or tip of one finger with up to two pounds of gentle force. Usually, just by lightly touching these points, you will know if they are painful. These points must not be just tender but must be painful on touch.

These tender points are painful specific sites in muscles, ligaments, tendons, and other soft tissues of the body. In some of these tender places, you will be able to feel nodules or tight bands that feel like a firm lump or "knot." Other painful spots are at insertion points of muscles into tendons and bones. Often the painful sites move around and can be related to muscle spasms. That is one reason to remove the tender point testing to confirm the fibromyalgia diagnosis.

In the research study, the most common area of pain was in the neck and shoulders area; 70% of participants indicated pain in the neck area, and 80% of the participants report pain in the shoulder area. The second most common area was the lower back where 72% indicated chronic pain. These numbers are in direct correlation to the numbers found by the American Academy of Pain Management. (NFCPA). They list the frequency of pain in the tender points to be found most commonly in the shoulders (84%), upper back (74%), knees (74%), lower back (62%), elbow area (62%), and neck (56%).

Hypersensitivity to Pain

The pain of fibromyalgia can vary between deep muscular aching, throbbing, burning, shooting and stabbing pains. Often, the pain and stiffness are worse in the morning. Once simple movement gets circulation to the muscles, the pain may decrease. Often, pain may be worse in the muscle groups used repetitively. The health of the nervous system can also affect the pain response in the body. Neuropathy is a term that describes nerve disease or injury. The most common type of neuropathy is a pinched nerve creating pain often with numbness. The deep spinal muscles cause the nerves to feel pinched. The term myofascial dysfunction describes muscle and tendon pain with neuropathy. "Myo" refers to muscle, and "fascia" refers to the connective tissue of muscle and tendon. Together, myofascial pain and neuropathy affect muscle dysfunction that leads to various patterns of acute or chronic pain.

Muscle spasms and chronic contraction of muscle fibers can come from this supersensitivity in the nervous system tissue. These spasms do not go away until restoration of nerve function. Chronic muscle contractions explain why a person with a low back pinched nerve has trouble with hamstring tightness and cannot bend over. As muscles remain persistently spastic or in a contracted position, they will eventually shorten and become tight causing abnormal joint movement and compression. Persistent contractions lead to abnormal wear points in the joints and cause pain in the connective tissues.

Since 2001, there have been a variety of research studies showing that people with fibromyalgia are truly more hypersensitive to pain. (Zareba, 2008, Dec). When the nerves in the muscle tissue become damaged, the reaction of the central nervous system is amplified, and hypersensitivity to pain occurs. The neurotransmitter that can cause the hypersensitive response is gamma-aminobutyric acid (GABA.) GABA is the primary inhibiting neurotransmitter that calms and stabilizes the brain. When people are sensitive to noises, odors, or pain, it is related to GABA imbalances.

Relationship with Other Diseases and Syndromes

The number and locations of tender points help to define fibromyalgia according to the American College of Rheumatology; yet, many other symptoms and conditions relate to fibromyalgia. (Jones, 2014). The most common associated symptoms are chronic fatigue, low-grade fever, swollen lymph nodes, anxiety, and depression. Other associated symptoms are:

1. A weakened immune system with chronic sore throats and swollen neck glands
2. Recurring headaches or migraines
3. Irritable bowel syndrome including symptoms of digestive complaints such as abdominal bloating, cramps, episodes of diarrhea and constipation, and problems of malabsorption
4. Cold sensitivity, poor circulation, and heart palpitations
5. Sleep difficulties
6. Restless leg syndrome, lightheadedness, and dizziness
7. Dry skin, dry eyes, and dry mouth
8. Recurring bladder infections in women
9. Joint pain, tenderness, morning stiffness, and burning sensations
10. Numbness and tingling of hands and feet
11. Concentration problems and brain fog

Chronic fatigue often associated with fibromyalgia makes some patients incapable of performing normal activities. Even minor exertion aggravates pain and creates deeper episodes of fatigue, without a specific cause except for lack of quality sleep. This fatigue is feeling completely drained of energy. Many patients say that their arms and legs are so heavy they feel like concrete blocks. This fatigue also affects the cognitive ability in the brain to think clearly.

Headaches were common symptoms in participants in the research project. One participant said that her head pain feels like "brain freeze," similar to the pain that we get when we eat ice cream too quickly. However, she has that feeling of pain constantly. There are many types of headaches, including migraines and sinus congestion pressure. Headaches have multiple causes. Most headaches can be relieved with increased circulation to the neck and head area, liver detoxification, and by making sure the body is well hydrated.

Fibromyalgia often relates to poor, non-restorative sleep. Patients with the syndrome wake up in the morning more exhausted than when they went to bed. Any sleep issues may precipitate fibromyalgia. On the other hand, the syndrome itself may lead to poor sleep. Since most patients with fibromyalgia have a poor sleep pattern, it is difficult to know which came first, the syndrome or the sleeping problem. One fascinating research study, about lack of sleep, shows that average people kept awake for several days develop specific pain points similar to those found on patients with fibromyalgia. (Choy, 2015).

Digestive disturbances are also associated factors in fibromyalgia syndrome. A common condition called "leaky gut syndrome" is related to malabsorption problems. When foods do not digest properly, and the lining of the intestines becomes weakened, the food particles leak through the wall of the intestine. Irritable bowel syndrome is related to "leaky gut syndrome" where intestinal inflammation occurs because the nutrients are not adequately broken down and become toxic to the system. Symptoms such as bloating, flatulence, diarrhea, and constipation are signs that there are digestive malabsorption problems. Leaky gut syndrome is one of the leading causes of all auto-immune diseases, not just fibromyalgia.

The immune system is affected by a dysfunctional digestive system. Bacterial imbalances in the intestines often cause symptoms such as sinus congestion, sore throat, swollen glands, and lymph nodes. Many of these symptoms and conditions become systemic (affect the whole body), since they are part of the regeneration phase of the self-healing cycle.

Causes of Fibromyalgia Symptoms

In my research project, I was looking for viable reasons for fibromyalgia pain. Doctors in 2001 were not sure what caused this chronic pain syndrome even though it was diagnosed often. Most doctors thought the pain was psychological and recommended anti-depressants. Auto-immune diseases were relatively new. Now fibromyalgia is considered an auto-immune disease and is related directly to chronic fatigue syndrome. According to functional medicine, metabolic imbalances cause fibromyalgia pain and chronic fatigue. Now we also know that people with fibromyalgia are hypersensitive to pain due to a motor/sensory imbalance affecting the nervous system. Trapped emotions, limiting beliefs, and social reactions also create metabolic variations associated with most auto-immune conditions.

An increased level of chronic muscle tissue breakdown is a cause for aching pain, and fatigue. The onset of pain may be gradual or sudden depending on the healing ability of our body. Often symptoms may appear after a traumatic event or illness, or after a stressful life event. Traumatic experiences can cause injury to the nervous system sensors making the muscles more hypersensitive to any reaction. This nervous system hypersensitivity can precipitate the tenderness on light touch often found in fibromyalgia patients. Fibromyalgia may also be associated with changes in muscle metabolism, leading to decreased blood flow, fatigue, and diminished strength. Another factor that may cause fibromyalgia is a specific virus or bacteria, but no exact infectious agent is identified. No conclusive patterns have been identified to be responsible for fibromyalgia syndrome. A variety of physical stress, lifestyle conditions, and emotions and beliefs are the cause of the symptoms.

Balance Adrenal and Thyroid Hormones

The pituitary is a gland in your brain controlled by your hypothalamus. The hypothalamus is in charge of regulating the set points in your body, including your body temperature, weight, and blood pressure. The hypothalamus is often the cause of hot flashes as it increases your temperature to activate low estrogen levels. The hypothalamus tells the pituitary which hormones to secrete. Then the pituitary, also called the master gland, secretes several hormones to the thyroid and adrenal glands.

Blood tests often look at TSH (thyroid stimulating hormone) secreted by the pituitary to see how the thyroid is functioning. If the TSH level is too high, that indicates a hypothyroid, or a weak thyroid condition, because the thyroid is activated by the pituitary. If the TSH is low, or less than 0.03, that can indicate a hyperthyroid. Most people with fibromyalgia are more hypothyroid than hyperthyroid. Here are common symptoms of low thyroid function.

- ✓ Have cold hands or feet often
- ✓ Have thin hair or lose many hairs daily
- ✓ Frequently constipated

- ✓ Loss of eyebrow hair on outside edge
- ✓ Have dry skin
- ✓ Weak sex drive
- ✓ Weak memory and concentration
- ✓ Swollen hands or feet
- ✓ Tend to be depressed

The thyroid depends on having balanced adrenal glands. Symptoms of adrenal imbalance are:

- ✓ Panic attacks
- ✓ Feel tired and wired
- ✓ Get fatigued easily
- ✓ Recurring headaches
- ✓ Crave sugar
- ✓ Crave salt
- ✓ Get dizzy when rising
- ✓ Tired even after sleeping well
- ✓ Have trouble falling asleep or staying asleep all night
- ✓ Cannot concentrate

Balancing both the thyroid and adrenal glands will improve energy metabolism. The thyroid gland is affected by environmental chemicals and radiation. Certain minerals like iodine, zinc, and selenium help support thyroid hormone conversion from T4 (thyroxine) to T3. Kelp has these minerals in whole food form. The adrenals use many minerals to regenerate and need more minerals when under stress or when fatigued.

The adrenal glands are two organs that sit on top of each kidney. They are shaped like small pyramids and are about the size of walnuts. They help us respond to daily stress in our lives. Your adrenals work with the pituitary and the hypothalamus to secrete hormones to keep the effects of stress in check in the glandular system. The adrenal glands produce specific hormones in response to different levels of stress.

The inner part of your adrenal glands, called the adrenal medulla, secretes adrenalin and noradrenalin. These hormones increase when you experience acute stress such as anger and fear. They are the hormones that help you gain energy for quick responses like running, lifting or fighting. These hormones cause an immediate rush of ATP energy that supply the muscles. Adrenalin hormones create the adrenal response that can make you extraordinarily strong for a short period.

The adrenal cortex, on the outside portion of the adrenal gland, responds to chronic stresses. Two of the hormones the adrenal cortex manufactures are cortisol and aldosterone. Aldosterone works together with the kidneys to regulate the mineral balance in the body. The proper balance of minerals is critically important in a healthy stress response.

Under normal conditions, the adrenal glands have enough cortisol and aldosterone to respond when there is stress and more energy is needed. However, the adrenal glands can only take so much stress. When this level of adrenal stress increases, the adrenals respond by making all the cortisol and aldosterone that they can, releasing them, then make some more, release them, and so on. At first, this repetitive response creates adrenal stress, causing too much cortisol and aldosterone in the system. Your body will use up minerals quickly, and weight gain will occur more easily as the increased cortisol levels cause insulin resistance. (Wilson, 2001).

Adrenal stress comes from a prolonged release of adrenaline hormones, a chronic elevation of heart rate and muscle tension, and a decrease in blood flow to organs. Also, there is an increase in the retention of sodium, water and calcium, and a thickening of the blood. Adrenal stress will deplete minerals, reduce immune system health, and increase fat storage from increased cortisol build-up. When cortisol increases, it brings on symptoms of fatigue, irritability, hypoglycemia, night sweats, sugar cravings, binge eating, and mental confusion.

Eventually, the adrenals become fatigued due to chronic stress, lack of sufficient vitamins and minerals, not enough sleep, lack of exercise, poor bowel function or hypoglycemia. As adrenal stress continues, the adrenals become more fatigued, which causes changes in mood, weakness from a decrease in the ability to effectively create energy, more depressive and confused thinking and increased susceptibility to allergies.

As this adrenal stress continues, you become so tired that you "cannot take it anymore." You rest for a few days and feel well enough to try again, but then the cycle repeats itself. After a few months or years of chronic stress, the adrenal glands become weak. Even after resting they are unable to respond to stress in a reasonable manner. The most common clinical manifestation of this condition is chronic fatigue.

Other signs of weak adrenal function include overeating and weight gain, especially in the abdominal area. When the adrenals are failing, the result is weight loss, excessive loss of salt from the kidneys and abnormally low blood pressure. This condition is called Addison's disease and occurs more in females. Only by strengthening the adrenals through diet, nutritional supplements and emotional stress reduction exercises will the adrenal fatigue improve.

When you crave sugar, it is usually a sign of adrenal stress or overactive adrenals. When you crave salt more than sugar that is a sign of adrenal fatigue. Now you need to balance your minerals. Adrenal fatigue indicates that you require more minerals in your diet to regenerate energy in your body.

In the presence of exhausted adrenals, the immune system function becomes weak also. A weak immune system makes people more susceptible to a variety of infections. Always look for weak adrenal or thyroid glands when you tend to get "everything that is going around" since the immune system is fragile. For example, the incidence of autoimmune disease goes up in the presence of weak adrenals. When the adrenals become fatigued, the immune system is allowed to attack specific cells of the body as if they were foreign invaders.

Anyone who becomes exhausted after stress, and remains exhausted, should have his or her adrenals tested. Do cortisol testing for people who become exhausted for days after even slight exertion. By having the adrenals tested, you can see the level of adrenal stress or fatigue and can begin taking supplements to improve the imbalance. A relaxing massage helps to reduce stress, as well as other relaxation techniques such as meditation, and both will gradually enhance adrenal function. Also adding more minerals in your diet from vegetables or supplementation will help you rebuild your adrenals.

Recommendations to Improve Adrenal and Thyroid Function

1. Test your cortisol levels, usually four saliva tests done during the day, to show your changing cortisol levels. Imbalanced cortisol levels can explain why you are tired during the day or awake at night.

2. During a blood test, measure more than TSH for thyroid function. TSH, or thyroid stimulating hormone, shows how the pituitary is regulating the thyroid. Get your free T3 and T4 levels measured too, to see how these thyroid hormones are working. The T4 thyroxine hormone converts to T3, and imbalances cause fatigue.

3. Get a massage regularly, or do other relaxing activities, to calm your stress levels.

4. Make sure you are getting enough minerals found in vegetables in your diet. We will discuss the benefits of magnesium later to see how it increases energy metabolism by supporting the adrenals.

Stress Triggers

Recognize Stress

Every day we are affected by the environment where we live. The way we respond to this environment instigates the stress in our lives. Our relationships, our work environment, our diet and exercise program, and our habits, both good and bad, all create reactions that our nervous system needs to control - physically, emotionally, and mentally. Chronic worries, such as financial or relationship problems, subject the body to mental stress. For many people, taking a test is very stressful. Driving can also be very stressful. Other people don't get stressed by test taking or driving. Our perception of these events is what causes stress. Too much uncontrolled stress can create pain and chronic illness.

In the research study, the percentage of participants who listed an accident or trauma that triggered the fibromyalgia symptoms was 56%. Accidents or traumatic events activate the nervous system. If these events are not discharged, the effects of trauma stay in the body creating biochemical and nervous system imbalances. Unless the trauma is released, the stress continues to build up, creating chronic stress reactions. Thirty percent of the fibromyalgia participants indicated that a car accident or fall brought on the symptoms, while 12% listed emotional trauma, such as divorce, abuse, or death of a loved one, as the initiating factor. When the fibromyalgia seems to be caused by an infection or another disease, it is the result of the infection not entirely leaving the body and staying stuck in the organ tissues.

To reduce trauma, identify the incident that caused the trauma. Did you have an accident, surgery, relationship change, or mentally traumatic event happen? Where is this trauma showing up in your body? How has this event changed your life?

Stress Triggers create neurological reactions in specific organ tissues. To find stress triggers, we need to ask questions:

> When did the pain initially begin? If it is a chronic problem, when was the very first time you noticed it?
> Did something change or shift in your life just before the pain symptom began?
> Is there a specific event or memory connected to this symptom?

It is essential to find the event that triggers your pain, especially with chronic issues. We remember stressful events when we are reminded about them when parallel events occur. For example, I had a traumatic event happen on Super Bowl Sunday. Now every time Super Bowl Sunday returns in February, it is a stress trigger for that upsetting event, more than the actual calendar date when the event happened.

Identifying the first time the stress triggered your symptoms helps to understand how your body is trying to protect you or help you survive more easily. When you locate the area of pain and which part of the brain is reacting, you will understand the root cause of pain. You may find an emotion or belief that is related to this stress trigger that can be transformed. By removing the trapped emotion or belief, your corresponding pain can also be vanished.

Test for Dominant Side

Do you have most of your pain on one side of your body? Or do you have other symptoms showing only on one side of your body, like skin conditions or weakness? There is a test for dominant sides to help you understand more about what can be causing your symptoms.

Which hand do you clap with? Put your hands together to clap as you do at a concert. Which hand is on top when you clap? Or if you clap with both hands moving together, which one is doing the major action?

The way you clap your hands is one way to know what side is dominant energetically. For myself, I clap with my left hand on top. I am not left-handed and tend to do everything with my right side - writing, kicking, and even listening while on the phone. So what hand is on top when YOU clap? And is it different than the hand you use to write?

Why does this make a difference? The dominant side technique helps determine the cause of a stress reaction that is showing up on the left or ride side of your body. For example, if you have eczema only on one side of your body, you may have an emotional reaction such as loss of touch or contact with someone. An issue with one eye can show up as an inability to visually see someone who is not close by, or being afraid of losing someone. Who is this person? To figure out who this individual is, you can use this hand dominance test.

When your right hand is on top when clapping - you are energetically right dominant. Your Yang or male side is your right side, and if the symptoms are on your right side, it could be your perception of a life situation related to your husband or wife, business partner, or father. If the health issue is on your left side, your more Yin side, the situation could be with a child, pet, or mother.

When your left hand is on top when clapping - you are energetically left dominant. Your Yang or male side is your left side, and if the symptoms are on your left, you could be observing a life situation with your husband or wife, business partner, or father. If the health issue is on your right side, your more Yin side, the situation could be with a child or mother. (LifestylePrescriptions®.TV, 2018).

Any identified family member or business partner should not be blamed for your symptom. They played a role that affected your stress reaction in that event. They probably were dealing with their own stress in that instance, and your energetic compassion absorbed that stress. When you couldn't release it, the stress it created was stored in your tissues. Children often pick up the stress of their parents, and the remembrance of this stress creates habit patterns later in life.

Understanding the dominant side can help you discern more about your pain. Is your fibromyalgia pain mostly on one side? Or do you feel weakness on one side more than the other? Use this clapping test to discover more about your cause of stress.

Specific Organ Tissue and Relating Conflicts and Symptoms

Fibromyalgia means fibrous muscle pain, so you may think stress only affects muscle tissue, and we just have to look at muscle health to understand the root cause of pain. As you have read, fibromyalgia is a syndrome, so we have to pay attention to different organ tissues that have overlapping factors affecting your metabolism. The organ tissues that are affected by stress triggers related to fibromyalgia syndrome are striated muscles, fascia, motor nerves, thyroid ducts and gland, adrenal medulla and cortex.

Striated muscle is the type of skeletal muscle that is most affected in fibromyalgia. These striated muscles are fibrous, dense tissues that repeatedly contract and relax to allow our body to move. These flexible muscles help maintain posture, stabilize joints, and help produce body heat. The cerebral medulla part of the brain controls the striated muscles. This area is affected by our self-worth, our feelings of strength, and our ability to move the way we want. When striated muscles are under stress, there is tissue breakdown, muscle atrophy, and weak stamina. During the regeneration phase, there is muscle edema, swelling, nerve irritation, and pain. You will experience muscle twitching and spasms during a healing peak.

Fascia is the connective tissue surrounding and protecting muscle and nerve fibers. It is controlled by the midbrain that supports the movement of tissues and the cerebellum that helps protect us from threats. In the stress phase there is an increase in the size of the tissues, and then during regeneration, the swelling goes back to normal. Fascia bundles muscle and nerve fibers and protects other structures. Layers of fascia in muscles merge to form a tendon that attaches to bones as the periosteum. Continuous fibers form a fascial connection throughout our body that allows pain to travel from one area to another.

This connective tissue makes up 20% of our body mass. These fascial muscle connections group together and according to Dr. Jerry Tennant in his book "Healing is Voltage," they work like a battery pack. (Tennant, 2010). The fascia surrounding the muscles acts like a semiconductor moving energy throughout your body and helps pump fluid around your body. Regular movement is needed to keep the fascia flexible and hydrated.

Motor nerves transmit impulses from the brain and spinal cord directly to the muscles. The cerebral cortex brain tissue controls these motor nerves. The cerebral cortex is affected by paralyzing trauma experiences associated with social perception and choices we make in our lives.

Where is the pain located? Many of the fibromyalgia tender points are located in the upper back and neck area. When we have pain in a specific place, we can relate these symptoms to conflicts. Here are the cerebral medulla conflicts relating to common muscle pain areas of fibromyalgia: (LifestylePrescriptions®.TV, 2018)

> Cervical spine and neck – Do you have someone in your life that is a "pain in the neck"? Is there someone who makes you feel insignificant?
> Shoulders – Do you feel like you should be doing something more, or are you carrying a heavy burden?
> Elbows – Are you being unbendable in any way with your desires?
> Lumbar spine – Do you feel undervalued from too much pressure?
> Hip bone – Do you have trouble standing up against a dominant person in your life?
> Knee – Do you feel inflexible in moving forward in your life?

Use your dominant side result and correlate it to your main location of pain. You can discover how your perception of a relationship situation is affecting your health. By increasing our awareness of how stress, emotions, and beliefs shape our symptoms we can take responsibility and change our perception of our life situations.

The thyroid and adrenal organs also react to stress triggers found in fibromyalgia and create energy in the tissues. There are two different tissues in each of these organs that have varied functions.

The brain stem controls the thyroid gland tissue, and it relates to survival, metabolism, and the inability to grasp or get rid of an issue. When the thyroid gland is in the stress phase the thyroid enlarges, and there is a faster metabolism and nervousness. During the regeneration phase the thyroid goes into hypofunction at first along with inflammation, and as it completes healing, it functions normally again.

The cerebral cortex controls the thyroid excretory ducts, and it relates to social interactions. When the thyroid ducts are stressed, there is a feeling of fear and powerlessness. Do you have recurring thoughts of being out of control? Or do you play the "What if … " mental game fearing the worst is going to happen? This can affect the thyroid excretory ducts.

The inability to deal effectively with external stress commonly shows up in the thyroid ducts. When we are exposed to too many toxins continuously, it can affect the thyroid ducts and create a chronic stress and regeneration pattern. Under stress, the thyroid ducts become weak due to ulceration. During the regeneration phase, there is swelling, cysts, and the auto-immune reaction of Hashimoto's thyroiditis.

The cerebral medulla controls the adrenal gland cortex, and it relates to feelings of self-worth and performance. The conflict related to this external part of the adrenal gland is feeling like you are on the wrong path or direction in your life. During the stress phase, there is reduced cortisol function, feeling stress and fatigued at the same time, weakness, and high blood pressure. In the regeneration phase, there is increased cortisol function and thickening of the tissue, potentially creating an adrenal cyst.

The adrenal medulla is the internal part of the adrenal gland controlled by the brain stem. The conflict related to the adrenal medulla is feeling overwhelmed or sensations of unbearable stress and anxiety. In the stress phase, there are high adrenaline, norepinephrine, and dopamine levels, along with high blood pressure. During the regeneration phase, the hormones go back into balance to get back to normal function. (LifestylePrescriptions®.TV, 2018)

Clearing Conflicts Causing Pain

We hold psychological conflicts in our tissues that show up as symptoms. You just read that different brain areas process stress reactions associated with organs differently. Pain and stiffness are common reactions to specific conflict themes. What are your recurring thoughts?

Do you have thoughts about personal issues of self-worth and performance? We hold mental/emotional pain in our striated muscles related to the cerebral medulla layer in our brain. Remember that striated muscle stress shows up as problems with our ability to move and use our strength the way we desire.

Or do you feel more social pressure from other people? Our muscles can become nearly paralyzed from traumas we have experienced and have not released. We become devalued and feel like we don't have the strength to move forward in social relationships from imbalanced nerves in the muscle.

Or do you have more of a survival issue related to the inability to digest previous events that affect the fascia in your muscles? Fascia stress comes from holding on to old unresolved experiences. Using reframing experiences or emotional clearing techniques these conflicts can begin to move out of the body.

To help clarify these types of conflicts in your body I recommend paying attention to what is going on in your body when you feel the pain. Ask yourself –

➤ What are you doing physically with your body? How are you sitting, standing, moving, and holding yourself?

➤ What are you focusing on mentally? Are you rehashing an event until it becomes engrained in your muscles and can't get out? When we repeatedly focus on stressful events, they get stuck in our energy patterns and affect the physical tissues.

➤ What are your beliefs about your pain? Are you able to get past this trauma or event, or don't you believe it is possible?

➤ What are you saying to yourself? Are you self-talking to yourself in a positive, encouraging way, or in a way that degrades you?

It takes practice, but it is worth it to find your own encouraging words and new beliefs. Once you answer these questions, you will have some direction of ways to improve your root cause of stress in your life. These behaviors can create stuck energy patterns in muscles, nerves, and other connective tissues. Here is an example of stress triggers showing up as pain reactions:

> *One of my clients had a customer service position that was going well until she had a new manager. This manager had her do 8 hours of repetitive motion daily for months, and over time she injured her neck, to the*

point that it showed up on an MRI and was diagnosed by a neurologist. She tried to tell this manager about her pain, but he dismissed it until she had so much nerve pain radiating from her neck to her hands that she couldn't lift anything. She was put on light duty at work, but the pain did not resolve as expected. She did see a chiropractor and did nutritional and homeopathic supplements that only helped minimally. We looked for psychological trauma being held in her tissues. She felt unheard and unappreciated for all of her work through her suffering. This shows up as a conflict in the cervical neck area.

Her nervous system was also reacting with tingling pain and weakness in her arms because she was looking for a new position and couldn't find one. Nerve pain comes from continued social trauma. When she did find a new job, within one week, her nerve pain was gone, and most of her neck pain was also better.

Then three months into her new position, there was a conflict between two of her bosses. She was told that she did her project wrong, even though it was correct according to the other boss. Her nerve pain returned, so her body remembered this stress response and reacted similarly. Once the boss's conflict was resolved, and she knew she was doing her best job, her pain settled down again.

Look at your current symptoms and the organ tissue conflict to confirm the areas you need to support. Also, review your Fibromyalgia Pain Quizzes results to see if you have thyroid or adrenal stress to monitor. Your metabolism is affected by all of these organ tissues, and balancing them with the following recommendations will move you through the regeneration phase more quickly.

Recommendations to Reduce Daily Stress

1. Live in the moment. Do not dwell on the past or worry about the future. Live by actively participating in the "now."

2. Keep a positive attitude in all activities as much as possible. Avoid complaining. What you focus on expands. Focus on being optimistic and grateful.

3. Plan your daily activities. Set expectations of what you want to happen in events in your life. Don't be rigid on making them happen, but have a direction to where you are progressing.

4. Get help to clear your recurring thought patterns. Talk to a Lifestyle Prescriptions® Health Coach to find specific actions that will release this trapped energy.

Emotions

Recognize Emotional Causes

Fibromyalgia has a strong emotional element. Twelve percent of the participants in the research study believe that emotional trauma was the initial cause of their fibromyalgia. More than 50% of the participants believe that stress from their work or personal life makes the fibromyalgia pain worse. The emotions from the initiating trauma or everyday stress become trapped in the muscle tissues and, when held for some time, constricts the muscles. Some of the common emotions that relate to fibromyalgia are feelings of resentment and hopelessness from work, family stress, or childhood memories.

Why do trapped emotions cause pain? One theory is that people with fibromyalgia have a lower pain threshold due to increased sensitivity of the brain's pain signals. Emotions are labels we give to energetic feelings we experience in our body. As we experience these feelings, nerves in our brain are consistently stimulated and increase the neurotransmitters that can create pain reactions. And there is a memory component. The pain receptors in the brain develop a memory of the pain that produces a consistent overreaction to pain signals. By looking at an MRI of the brain, increased regional brain blood flow in the primary motor area is seen in people with fibromyalgia. This increased activity can produce problems in processing pain signals.

Our emotions and experiences are essentially energy stored in the cellular memory of our bodies. Do you have recurring pain in one area of your body? It is likely this location in your body still holds energy from that experience. When you have a pain in certain areas, it's often related to something emotional you are feeling within yourself. We don't realize this because we are so busy taking care of others that we don't have time to think about our issues. We ignore our symptoms until they demand attention by creating pain responses.

Take time to feel your own emotions, and where they are in your body. Look at both negative and positive emotions. When you feel a specific pain, what energy or emotion is stuck in that tissue right now? And how strong is it on a scale of 1 to 10? Then, think back and remember if there is a time that this emotion was stronger, or when it first began. You can also look for an underlying emotion. We often can identify a surface layer emotion. There are intense emotions, four or more layers deep that make up the real core emotion. Strong emotions help you figure out how the conflicts in our body affect our emotional health. Think about the organ experiencing pain, the stress trigger for the pain, and conflict associated with the organ tissue to help you find the underlying emotions. As you will see here, negative emotions affect how our organs function.

The limbic system in our brain becomes oversensitive to pain due to chronic thoughts of pain and experiences related to the pain. The more often you experience physical, mental, or emotional pain, the more nervous system reactions you will have when re-thinking about the pain. After injuries create pain impulses, our body should be able to counteract the pain during recovery of the nervous system. The recalling of painful experiences indeed increases our sensitivity to it and will overload your ability to let go of physical pain. Recalling painful experiences is a conditioned reflex that is often the cause of chronic pain responses.

There may be inherited emotional energy that is affecting you. Often we can inherit emotions and energy patterns from parents or grandparents when they have unresolved issues. Are you named after a relative? Can you find out more about their life and what mental and physical health issues they had? Generational family issues can linger in children until the emotion or unresolved issue is recognized and fixed.

Emotions held in our body often create physical imbalances. Any chronic emotion such as fear, anger, hostility or sadness will cause the adrenal glands to secrete cortisol. When cortisol elevates for any length of time, it will affect the behavior of specific organs. Hardening of the arteries and cancer are two examples of significant causes of death that can be related to increased cortisol levels. Also, obesity is another problem related to excess cortisol levels. Excessive cortisol can cause gradual weight gain, especially in the abdominal area.

The immune system requires adequate levels of cortisol to function properly. We do need a certain amount of stress in our lives as stimulation for us to perform effectively. Of course, what constitutes an adequate level of stress varies from person to person. Excessive cortisol can speed up the immune system dangerously causing adrenal stress.

For example, if you feel anger, yet you ignore it, soon you will find an elevation of anger in many other areas of your life. Eventually, you'll believe that everyone is against you. Your body continues to secrete cortisol to make immune antibody cells to counteract all this pent up emotion. You will become more prone to chronic fatigue, and chronic colds or immune weakness. Ultimately, you may have many excess antibodies that turn against each other causing autoimmune diseases.

Alternatively, your body can also become so tired of these negative excess emotions that you will be physically and emotionally exhausted of this struggle. Then your body will stop producing cortisol and immune cells. As these levels decrease, the body becomes chronically depressed and adrenal fatigue develops. The body's minerals become exhausted from continually trying to fight these emotions, and the immune system becomes worn out. In this state, susceptibility to infections, and sensitivities to environmental chemicals increase, while the lack of necessary energy to heal well, is not available.

Positive emotions are important to realize as part of the healing program. To engage in new positive habits, it is beneficial to focus on positive emotions. What emotion do you want to feel in creating your new healthy habit? Some powerful positive emotions are joy, gratitude, love, peace, trust, and appreciation.

Too often we focus on negative emotions we experience. When we focus on positive emotions and become more positive in general, we will truly have more positive experiences. A happy mindset is a positive mindset. Do you have feelings of contentment or happiness in your life? By choosing more positive thoughts to control your actions, you will have more encouraging interactions. Enjoy your daily journey. We never achieve happiness; it only exists in the present moment.

Chinese Medicine and Emotions

In Chinese medicine, certain emotions relate to certain organs. Chinese medicine also links organs into five elements called Fire, Earth, Metal, Water, and Wood.

➢ The heart connects with the fire element, and its associated negative emotions are overwhelmed and confusion. The positive emotions are joy and happiness.

➢ The spleen and stomach are associated with the earth element, and with the emotions of anxiety and worry. Anxious thoughts about the future create immune system stress by affecting the spleen.

➢ The lungs and large intestine equate with the metal element and associate with grief and conflict.

➢ The kidney and bladder work together in the water element and emotionally are related to insecurity and restlessness.

➢ The liver and gall bladder are related to the wood element and emotionally are associated with anger and resentment. For example, when anger becomes chronic, the liver physically enlarges, and the many functions of the liver are affected.

Recognizing your recurring emotions will enable you to identify the type of stress you may be inflicting on your organs.

Specifically, according to Chinese Medicine, the symptoms of fibromyalgia have been linked most often to liver, gallbladder, and spleen meridian imbalances. The liver meridian stores and cleanses the blood, and maintains the flow of energy that controls the flexibility of the muscles, ligaments, and tendons. When the liver energy is deficient, dryness occurs in the skin and tendons, and blood flow in the body is restricted. Also, liver imbalances bring on symptoms of frustration, irritability, and feeling stuck; and commonly produce an emotional state of constant resentment, with repressed anger or depression. (Beinfield, 1992).

The gallbladder meridian is the source of courage and initiative and is responsible for decision-making. Physically, the gallbladder meridian controls the circulation of the energy that protects and nourishes the cells, and when out of balance weakens the ligaments and tendons. Symptoms of insomnia, wandering pains, weakness in the legs and chest, and side pains come from gallbladder weakness.

The spleen meridian governs digestion, and imbalances manifest in the muscles. The spleen meridian also relates to feelings of stability, including feeling centered and balanced. The excessive use of the mind tends to weaken the spleen meridian energy flow. Mental stress comes from excess emotional worry or anxiety about the future. Imbalance in the spleen meridian energy flow manifests as morning fatigue, craving for sweets, nausea, flatulence, loose stools, pale lips, swelling of the abdomen, and muscular weakness.

Emotions may not seem significant and may be easy to ignore in your daily life. Research shows that it takes 6 hours for your immune system to recover from a quick negative emotional experience. On the other hand, when we have an encouraging emotional experience, there is an immediate increase in beneficial chemicals that have a positive effect on the immune system. For example, when we feel loved or appreciated and remember it, nourishing chemicals are released into our immune system.

When we make positive statements, instead of negative statements, our immune system is enhanced. Even our thoughts, whether positive or negative, will affect our immune system. Having a critical temperament towards yourself and others will create more immune system problems than having a positive temperament. Sometimes we are more critical of ourselves than we are of others. Remember always to treat others like you would want to be treated, and treat yourself like you want others to treat you.

Here's a story demonstrating how unresolved emotions can cause physical pain.

A few years ago, a relative called me with constant low back pain that began after being out of town for the weekend. She went to her medical doctor, and he could not find anything that could be causing it. Medication did not help. Then she went to a chiropractor, and his treatment made the pain worse. Eventually, she called me to send her a homeopathic remedy to relieve the pain. I found a remedy that matched her physical symptoms. She took a few doses of the remedy the next day, and her pain went away. While talking about the quick relief from pain, I asked what, if anything, happened in her life just before this pain started. She remembered that only a couple days before the pain began, she had argued with her husband. This argument didn't get resolved before she went out of town.

This story is an example of emotional constipation when low back pain comes from not letting go of conflict. She was physically holding on to this conflict in her lower back, which according to Chinese Medicine theory is a common place to hold unresolved issues. Homeopathic remedies work on physical and emotional symptoms and often help resolve this type of emotional difficulty along with physical symptoms. Homeopathic remedies that are commonly used for fibromyalgia, to relieve both physical and emotional pain, will be explained in a later section.

Emotions are often related to underlying limiting beliefs. In the next section, we will look at how creating new empowering beliefs will help release trapped emotions.

Recommendations to Improve Emotional Imbalances

1. Realize that trapped emotions can be causing your pain symptoms. Become aware of where you feel emotions in your body. Go to the

area of pain at the moment, and feel the emotion you are holding there. It may take some time at first, yet soon you will be able to recognize your emotions. Then it is easier to shift them with emotional clearing techniques

2. Use a list or chart of emotions to help identify which emotions you have. There are general emotions like fear, anger, and grief. More complex charts are available to find more specific emotions. I use the Emotion Code technique with my clients to release held emotions. This procedure uses an emotion chart and muscle testing to identify emotions. Then using a simple magnetic energy process, you can release each emotion. You can identify when the emotion occurred, where it is in your body, and if another person is involved in the emotion when doing the Emotion Code technique. (Nelson, 2007)

3. Make sure to find a positive emotion to replace the negative emotions so that you can focus on a new emotional pattern. Bring more joy, gratitude, peace, love, inspiration, confidence, appreciation, and enthusiasm into your life depending on what resonates with you. Happiness is only found in the present moment. Realize the experiences that bring contentment into your life.

4. Learn EFT (Emotional Freedom Technique) that uses tapping on certain points on your head and upper body, along with direct phrases to help unblock the stuck emotion. There are five steps to EFT tapping you can repeat until you feel relief. (Ortner, 2013)

A. Identify the issue – Find the issue or emotion you are having, and where it is in your body. Do only one issue at a time.

B. Test the initial level of intensity of pain on a scale of 1 to 10. Make ten the highest worst intensity. Identifying the initial intensity helps set a benchmark for future reference.

C. Then, create a setup phrase you want to address. Identify the issue and accept yourself as complete even though you have this problem. The common phrase used is "Even though I have this (emotion in this organ tissue), I deep and completely accept myself."

D. Go into the EFT tapping sequence on the end of 9 Chinese meridian points:

1. Karate chop point on pinky finger side of hand - small intestine meridian.
2. Between the eyebrow – bladder meridian
3. Outside of eye – gall bladder meridian
4. Under the eye – stomach meridian
5. Under the nose – governing vessel
6. Middle of the chin – central vessel
7. Between the beginning of the collarbone and the sternum – kidney meridian
8. Under the arm – spleen meridian
9. Top of head – governing meridian

Begin by tapping on the karate chop point by saying your setup phrase three times. Then tap each point 7 times, moving down the head and body in order. Finish each round tapping on the top of your head. While tapping the points in order, you can shorten your phrase to remind yourself of the organ tissue, stress trigger, and emotion. (LifestylePrescriptions®.TV, 2018). Say, for example – "I release this pain in my neck." "I release this emotion of fear." Go through the 9 points 3 times, with the final time bringing in the new positive emotion you want to feel instead. "I feel joy," or "I feel confident," or whichever one you desire.

E. Test the final intensity level on a scale of 1 to 10. If you don't get it to go down low enough repeat the process until you feel relief. Many people see very positive results with the Emotional Freedom Technique. There are great books and training available to help you learn more about it. https://www.healthline.com/health/eft-tapping#treatment

Beliefs

You don't manifest what you want; you manifest what you believe. A belief is a feeling of certainty about what something means. We create beliefs based on our past pleasurable or painful experiences. But the past doesn't have to predict our future or our present. I like this quote by Eleanor Roosevelt. "Yesterday is history. Tomorrow is a mystery. Today is a gift. That is why they call it the present."

Beliefs are repetitive thoughts we believe to be true. Be mindful of your unconscious tape player in your mind showing up as recurring thoughts. We can change our present state by taking action toward the results we want, not the results we got in the past. When you see different results from new activities, you will create new beliefs.

When we have unrealized goals in our life, we often have recurring thoughts that are limiting our success. These are belief patterns that hold us back from our potential. We know we should make healthier food choices, but we go back to old patterns too easily. Why is that? It could be a belief we are telling ourselves. When we don't get the results we want, we most likely have unconscious beliefs that help sabotage our good intentions.

If we believe something will not work out for us, even unconsciously, we will not take action, and prove that our belief is true. Beliefs can help us move forward, or hold us back. Beliefs give us certainty about our decisions since change is not always really wanted. We like our comfort zone, and often belief patterns keep us there. Most of our beliefs are unconsciously created based on our perceptions and interpretations of experiences in our past. We often look for experiences to back up our ideas. You can change limiting beliefs to empowering beliefs.

Common limiting beliefs –

> ➢ I am not good enough, or smart enough.
> ➢ I am not worthy.
> ➢ I don't deserve love.
> ➢ I don't have time.
> ➢ I am too old, or too young.
> ➢ I don't have willpower.
> ➢ It's too expensive to eat well.
> ➢ My family has chronic pain, so it runs in my family. I will have chronic pain too.

We find experiences to back up our limiting beliefs. The key to change is to be aware of our beliefs, and then change them into empowering beliefs.

Beliefs can change quickly or slowly. When we have low expectations, we don't believe change is possible, and we will tend to have chronic fibromyalgia pain. To make changes you can write out your limiting beliefs, and then ask yourself four questions. These questions help reframe your beliefs to be more empowering:

1. Is this belief true?
2. Is this belief true 100% of the time? When is it not true?
3. How do you react when you believe that thought? Is there an emotion related to it?

4. Who would you be without this belief? How would your life be different? How would you feel without this belief? Turn the belief around to experience the opposite. And find at least two specific examples of how each turnaround is right in your life.

Learn to visualize your ideal scenario with you living your new positive belief. Use encouraging statements in the present tense to ingrain these positive visualizations in your head. My two favorite statements begin:

"I am so happy now that I can (move easily and without pain.)"
"I am so grateful that I am now (able to travel again to visit my family.)"

I added examples to these statements of potential positive beliefs you may desire. Put your own specific words in the parentheses. Twice per day visualize yourself moving freely again, with confidence, while saying these statements to ingrain this new belief in your limbic system.

Values

Beliefs are what you accept as true, while values express what is important in your life. Values and beliefs do change as we move through life. Our beliefs can show up in the expectations of our self and others. So pay attention to what you think should happen in any situation. Your expectations will help lead you to your values. Values determine your priorities, and we often measure our happiness in life on how well we are harmonizing our values.

To find your current values ask yourself - "What is important to me?" I like to use some of Dr. John DeMartini's questions from his book "The Values Factor" to elicit values. (DeMartini, 2013). The questions I often ask are:

1. What do you love to do?
2. What do you love to learn about most?
3. How do you fill your space in your home?
4. How do you spend your time?
5. How do you spend your energy?
6. How do you spend your money?
7. What do you most often talk to yourself about?
8. What do you most often talk to others about?

Make a list of 10 different values and then put them in order of most important to least important to you. Typical values are love, integrity, honesty, happiness, health, reliability, prosperity, family, freedom, independence, dependability, compassion, success, acceptance, and fairness. You may discover many other values within you.

1. _____
2. _____
3. _____
4. _____
5. _____
6. _____
7. _____
8. _____
9. _____
10. _____

To prioritize your values, see if there is a common theme and group those together. Then decide which value overrides another value. For example, is health important to you? Is it more important than your family? If your family is more important to you than your health, then you will prioritize your time for family issues, and maybe forego health improvement until you have more time. Sometimes there are values conflicts. Often these are seen between career and family priorities. Do you ever feel guilty making time for work responsibilities over time for children? Working mothers have this value conflict often. Understanding and staying congruent in your values is essential.

<u>Top 5 Values by Priority</u>

1. _____
2. _____
3. _____
4. _____
5. _____

Also listen for negative values or values you want to avoid. Some common negative values are hostility, regret, anxiety, rejection, embarrassment, jealousy, failure, judgment, frustration, guilt, greed, and depression. Do you first think of these types of values in your daily thoughts? By recognizing values you want to avoid, you can find the opposite positive value. For example, no one likes rejection. To turn that around, what value do you want to bring into your life? More acceptance?

Discover your top 5 positive values and then look back in your life and remember times when you experienced your highest values. What were you doing to represent your value? Who were you with at that time? What factors contributed to this feeling? Look for similar value events in your daily life that can nourish you.

It is important once you find your values to be congruent with them. When we are not congruent, we feel guilt or shame because we are not living the life we expect. For fibromyalgia, you may feel you can't live up to your values due to your chronic pain and fatigue. That is one reason health needs to be a significant value for you. Do you remember a time when you felt like you were healthy? What were you doing? What was important at that time? How do you want health to show up in your life? What would be your ideal state to express health? Focus on that feeling and bring more of it into your life.

Many of life's decisions are really about determining what you value most. By becoming aware of your values, you will understand yourself better. When making decisions, you can rely on your values as the guiding force to go in the right direction. Identifying your particular values can take time and be a challenging, yet worthwhile, exercise.

Social

Relationships

The way we interact with family and friends, and our environment, affects our metabolism and potentially our pain responses. Having good supportive relationships helps in the healing process. When we are in pain, we often do not want to participate in activities, and our social life will suffer. It is vital to identify those special people you can rely on to be there when you need support. Also, even when you don't feel well, due to too much pain or fatigue, it is best to stay as optimistic as possible. Make specific plans on ways you can interact with family and friends regularly. Social interaction is needed especially for mental health.

Do you talk about your symptoms to others? Why do you do that? Often we are looking for support by engaging others in our experiences. Getting support from others is a way to meet our own human needs. Psychologist Chloe Madanes and Tony Robbins help people discover how they are fulfilling their six human needs. In their Core 100 coaching program, they teach Human Needs Psychology to describe the basic needs we all try to meet in our lives. (Robbins, 2017). We try to fill the needs that are most important to us either consciously or unconsciously. We can fill these needs in either a positive or a negative way. When we try to fill these needs in ways not aligned with our values, we will encounter conflicts. When we meet our needs in align with our values, we will be satisfied. The six basic needs are:

1. Certainty – the need for security and stability. Knowing we are right.
2. Variety – the need for change and challenges.
3. Significance – the need to be accepted, valued and acknowledged.
4. Love and connection – the need to feel loved and supported by others
5. Growth – the need to continue learning and developing new skills
6. Contribution – the need to help others, giving our time to make a difference.

The first four human needs are physical needs, and the last two human needs are spiritual needs. Most people find that two of the first four needs are more important than the other two. Do you crave certainty so much that you don't like change? Or do you tell people your fibromyalgia story to gain connection? Or significance? Sometimes we look for ways to be acknowledged when we have pain so that we get confirmation that we are vital to others. Acknowledgment is okay depending on your reason. Are you trying to justify your pain, so you don't have to take action to improve it? Or are you looking for social support to help you feel more positive and connected?

Take some time and think about each of these needs, and how you are meeting these needs in your life right now. Are you meeting your needs positively or negatively? Also, in your social situations, you can watch how other people are meeting their own needs too. Noticing other family and friend's needs can be a fascinating exercise. Your social life will improve as you understand yourself and recognize your family's needs.

Another social element that often can create nervous system stress showing up as pain is giving priority to caring for others over your own self-care. I see clients that put all their energy into their family's needs, ignoring their own needs. You just looked at your individual needs. Did you find that you thought that your needs are not as important as your children's needs? Or are you taking care of aging parents, and you have extra responsibilities to be there for them? It is essential to be there for others, but not at the expense of your health. Your family needs you to be healthy and strong so that you can be a positive force for others too. Young mothers of multiple children constantly are mediating issues and conveying important principles daily. By showing your children and the rest of your family how you take care of yourself, you will set a great example.

Recommendations to Reduce Social Stress

➢ According to responses by participants in the research study, many people hold long-term chronic stress from work or relationships that cause "lack of control" thoughts. We can't always be in control, especially if we work for someone else. We can decide to keep a positive attitude instead of complaining all the time. We can bring control into our lives by creating beneficial habits that create certainty. When we know we can use specific techniques to be in control of our lives; we store less stress.

➢ Having a sense of purpose or passion will create significance and a way to contribute to the world. I find when people know why they do something, even if its not their favorite thing to do, it becomes less stressful. Do you know what you want? Why are you doing the job or career you have chosen? Knowing that you are progressing in a positive direction is helpful. Going with the flow of the crowd (or your family) usually doesn't help in the long term to reduce mental stress. Write down what you desire in your life – positive things that will move you forward.

➢ Reduce social stress by managing your expectations of yourself and others. Sometimes we create unrealistic goals for ourselves; and then when we don't attain them, we have the beliefs that we are not good enough, or deserving. With relationships, we can have expectations of others that are impractical. Whether it is for your expectations or others, make sure you are clear on what you want or expect to happen. Communicate with others what you are anticipating. A common issue in relationships is predicting that the other person knows what we want. It may be challenging to speak up with your expectations, but ultimately, it will make your relationships better. People can't read our mind, and when we hope that they will do something, we must tell them. Clarity is valuable when we know what we want and then express it to others.

➢ Create supportive connections with friends and family that care about you. Who is in your circle of trusted friends? When you have chronic work stress and you can't talk to your boss about it, then having a confidant that will listen is needed. You can also work with a Lifestyle Prescriptions® Health Coach that will be there to listen to your needs, and enhance your understanding of your actions, thoughts, beliefs, and values.

Environmental

A social factor to reduce fibromyalgia symptoms is to increase your ability to release toxins. We are exposed to many toxins daily, not just from the environment, but also from metabolic wastes we create. Wastes build up inside our cells creating a toxic environment if not released. Toxins slow elimination and circulation. Muscle pain comes from these toxins creating congestion. To get rid of congestion pain we need to increase flow and clear the path for the removed toxins. Toxins stop our tissues from absorbing and using nutrients.

In the United States, we import or produce 74 billion pounds of chemicals every year. We get exposed to about 250 different types of chemicals each day. And this number is increasing by 3% each year. (EPA, 2010). By 2024 we will double the number of chemicals we live with daily. Plus only about 5% of them are proven safe. Many of these chemicals are plastics, food additives, household cleaners, solvents, paints, flame retardants, and pesticides. They get into our body through our skin, by inhaling the chemicals in the dust, and by ingesting them.

Why do chemicals affect our metabolism so much? Their structure is similar to our thyroid hormone, our primary metabolic hormone, so chemicals are an endocrine disrupter. (Meeker, 2012). The chemicals attach to our cells and are absorbed where the hormones are supposed to work. They affect how everything works in our body, not just our hormones. Chemicals affect our nervous system, changing how we make energy and how we think.

Food additives are increasing by 10% each year in our processed foods. That is why I read all labels of the foods I buy. I look for foods with less than four ingredients, and none of them can have high fructose corn syrup, MSG, food colorings, gums or yeast extracts. These are abundant in most processed foods, and usually, indicate that other chemicals are also in that food. Even foods with "natural flavors" listed can have chemicals we need to avoid. Reduce chemicals from your diet first, and you will make a big difference. One study showed that eating unprocessed organic foods lowered the number of pesticides measured in children's bodies by over 50% in only 15 days. (EWG, 2015)

Chemicals bind to our cells and do not release well. They build up in tissues. Toxins change the protein molecules in our cells. It makes it look like a foreign cell. Then our immune system reacts to stop this different cell from working. All of the common chronic diseases are related to environmental toxin buildup from foods or chemicals.

Pesticides and plastics are the nasty toxins, and we can't underestimate reactions they create. Other common toxins are mold, heavy metals, and BPA ink on receipts that bind to our hormone receptors and change how we absorb hormones and create auto-immune reactions. Heated plastics in our take-out coffee cups and acidic soft drinks make the plastic from the container get into cells. Styrofoam cups release toxins after heating the coffee or tea. Teflon pots are easy to use but terrible for our hormones. More to consider are skin care and antibacterial products, including body washes. Dial soap in the late 1940s came out with deodorant soap that smelled great. But it had a chemical called hexachlorophene that was banned by the FDA in 1971 due to reactions in blood. Triclosan is a pesticide used in antibacterial soap since 1980. Now, triclosan is prohibited by the FDA because of auto-immune reactions. As discussed earlier, our thyroid is very susceptible to imbalances when excess toxins are in the environment.

Read ingredients in all of your personal care products. If you are a hairdresser or painter, you may have more toxins. Many lipsticks use lead to hold the color on our lips. Don't ignore symptoms you have after using any products. Common symptoms of a runny nose, tingling or numbness, headaches, congestion, or low-grade fever are signs of toxic reactions.

Common toxins also come from remodeling projects in our home like new paint, carpeting, and vinyl products. Excess home air pollution and exhaust from cars are also the cause of other common issues like obesity, cardiovascular symptoms, allergies, and asthma. All these toxins knock out our mitochondria and stop our energy production. When we have weak energy pathways, our immune system can't fight off bacteria, viruses, and allergens.

Our liver will store excess toxins in our fat cells. When people lose weight, they can have reactions to releasing toxins. That is one reason it is so important to drink enough water when losing weight. Headaches are common detox symptoms caused by not drinking enough water. Find the cause, and change your diet or use of toxins so that your liver can begin to release built-up toxins.

Fibromyalgia pain comes from the gradual accumulation of toxic chemicals in the soft tissues, especially in areas where we tend to hold stress, such as the neck, shoulders, and lower back. Any place where toxins build up in the tissues, the blood becomes thicker, slowing down circulation, and slowing down healing. The accumulation of toxic chemicals, lack of circulation, and the lack of oxygen all lead to sluggishness in the lymph system. When the lymph fluid becomes stagnant, it causes the lymph nodes to swell and become sore. The pain in the tender points relates to this buildup of toxic lymph tissue in these areas. Insufficient oxygen in any cell of the body interferes with the healing process. A natural consequence of too little oxygen is the build-up of lactic acid, causing soreness in these hypersensitive areas of tender points.

There are two principal ways that chemical toxins enter the body and get into the blood. They come in as a result of what we eat and breathe. At first, the body will reject toxins. When we cough or sneeze, or when we vomit after eating contaminated foods, our body is trying to eliminate toxins. But over time, especially when these toxic chemicals are introduced into our tissues in tiny amounts over time, the blood and organs get weakened, and the toxins build up in the tissues.

How do you know if you have toxic imbalances? You can understand by the intensity of the symptoms you have in the following areas:

Digestive symptoms:

- bad breath
- gas and bloating
- heartburn
- constipation or diarrhea
- foul odor to the stool
- food allergies
- tired after meals

Respiratory symptoms:

- sinus congestion
- ear congestion
- recurring bronchitis
- asthma attacks

Nervous system symptoms:

- loss of concentration or memory
- anxiety
- irritability
- excessive worry
- coordination problems

- o depression

Circulatory symptoms:

- o headaches or migraines
- o arthritis
- o cold hands and feet
- o numbness or tingling
- o low back pain

Skin symptoms:

- o body odor
- o eczema or psoriasis

These toxic symptoms should last only a short time, as long as you do not suppress them. Just be aware of whenever you have these symptoms acutely, it can indicate a toxic reaction to something in your current environment.

Common symptoms that occur with an acute reaction to a food you just consumed are headaches, runny nose, or watery eyes. Another way to know if a substance causes your body to over-react is to measure your pulse. Coca's pulse test for food reactions begins by measuring your resting pulse for one minute. Then eat food you believe you may be sensitive to, or that you crave. Measure your pulse again after 30 seconds. When your pulse increases by more than 5 points after eating a single food, your nervous system is over-reacting to that substance.

Ideally, perform this Coca test with simple foods, not combinations like sandwiches or casseroles. When you realize after a meal that your heart is racing, take time to test every single ingredient in that meal every hour to find the culprit. Pay attention to your reactions to ingredients. You can make better decisions on foods when you know you will not feel right after eating certain kinds.

The Liver's Role in Cleansing

The liver is the main organ that is responsible for keeping the body clear of toxins. The liver uses minerals and enzymes to neutralize toxic chemicals. The liver has two steps, or phases, to eliminate toxins from the system. In phase 1, the liver uses an enzyme to oxidize, or remove, toxic chemicals from the blood. In phase 2, the liver changes the toxic chemicals into a water-soluble state that is easier to release from the tissues. When the detoxification phases of the liver are not working efficiently, then any toxic chemicals created by undigested food will cause more stress on the liver.

When the liver continues to use up all the minerals to suppress the toxic chemicals, it will become congested. Then the liver cannot carry out its metabolic functions as efficiently. Once the liver is over 70% congested, toxic chemicals collect in the blood and eventually in the connective tissues. The reaction to toxic chemicals in tissue creates acute symptoms such as excess mucus, skin conditions, and either diarrhea or constipation. Recognize these symptoms as the body's response to suppressed toxic chemicals.

When we are in a healthy state, the chemical toxins can be released through the system more quickly. Discharge of toxins can show up as an acute disease pattern. In this pattern, the toxins get released through the skin or the mucous membranes in the nose or throat. Maintaining good drainage is needed to get rid of recent toxic exposures.

When an acute toxin reaction is suppressed, by anti-histamines for example, the toxic chemicals build up in the cells creating chronic symptoms from an increased toxic state. The vitality of the body lessens, and it becomes even more difficult to remove the toxins. Once tissues become weak from a buildup of congestion, it is best to take smaller steps in the cleansing process.

Simple steps will assist in eliminating detoxifying reactions such as headaches and diarrhea. This weakened condition is called a chronic disease pattern. Most often we develop a weak chronic state from suppressing the acute cleansing reactions we just discussed. The body begins to become fatigued, and the vulnerable tissues degenerate from their normal function. Suppression of cleansing reactions initiates autoimmune diseases or syndromes such as chronic fatigue syndrome or fibromyalgia.

Microbes and the Brain Layers

Four brain relay connections relate to specific types of actions of the tissue supported by them. These are embryonic layers of the brain known as the endoderm, mesoderm, and ectoderm. They are related to the inner to outer brain development, and each area affects different tissue. The four brain areas associated with these embryonic layers are the brain stem, the cerebellum, cerebral medulla, and cerebral cortex. The brain stem is the oldest part of the brain, relating to the endoderm. The organ tissues controlled by the brain stem help with survival. The brain stem controls many of the digestive organs showing that strong digestion is related to survival.

The brain stem uses fungi and bacteria to help decompose tissues formed during the stress phase of healing. The organs most affected are the intestines, liver, kidney, and lung tissues. During the regeneration phase, the bacteria decompose excessive cell growth, and the waste is released. Yeast infections and candida, related to excess sugar in the diet, are the mycobacteria most often found in brain stem tissues.

The cerebellum is in the mesoderm part of the brain. The organ tissues related to the cerebellum are the dermis of the skin, muscle fascia, and myelin sheath. All these tissues help physically protect us from outside invaders. Conflicts related to cerebellum tissues relate to self-protection. Microbes associated with the cerebellum help us make sure we do not get attacked mentally and emotionally. Acne, abscesses, and melanoma are common dermis skin reactions showing the release of these bacteria. These are clean-up reactions moving the toxins out of deeper tissues.

The cerebral medulla is also in the mesoderm embryology layer. The organ tissues related to the cerebral medulla are muscles, bones, cartilage, and striated muscle tissues. Other tissues controlled by the cerebral medulla are the lymph tissue, spleen, and blood vessels. The conflicts related to cerebral medulla tissues relate to self-worth and performance. For example, when we don't feel strong mentally due to a stress reaction, we will create weakness in our muscles or bones. Certain types of bacteria help rebuild bones and muscles after stress reactions weaken them. The pneumonia bacteria is an example of a cerebral medulla regeneration microbe where fever and swelling occur as part of the healing process.

The cerebral cortex is in the ectoderm embryology layer, the youngest part of the brain. The organ tissues related to the cerebral cortex are the senses, digestive and endocrine ducts, and the mucous membranes. The cerebral cortex conflicts are related to social perceptions. When we feel powerless, or our territory or boundaries are not honored, we will have weakness in these tissues. Viruses come into the mucous membranes to reconstruct these tissues after ulceration, creating fever and inflammation reactions. Next time you have a viral infection, you can think of it as part of the regeneration phase of self-healing. (LifestylePrescriptions®.TV, 2018).

Microbial Infections

Microbes come from bacteria, viral, fungal, and parasite toxins. A build-up of toxins from microbes causes muscle spasms, stiffness, and hypersensitivity. There are many remedies to reverse these muscle and nervous system imbalances. The goal is to improve circulation and move toxins out of the body every day.

Usually, eighty-five percent of the bacteria in the colon is supposed to be the "good" or beneficial type of bacteria. In individuals with malabsorption problems, there is a definite increase in toxic bacteria. An imbalance of bacteria comes from the consumption of sugar and processed food, the use of steroid medications and aspirin, and stress. Symptoms of lower bowel gas, bloating, constipation, skin problems, chronic upper respiratory congestion, and undigested food in the stool, all indicate an imbalance of bacteria in the colon.

To assist in rebalancing the bacteria in the colon, use certain foods or supplements containing probiotics such as acidophilus. Many different types of beneficial bacteria help to reduce fungal and bacterial imbalances, lower cholesterol, improve the absorption of nutrients, and detoxify the colon of toxic bacteria.

If you get tired after meals, you can check for bacterial toxins in the intestine by changing your diet. For three days eat nothing with sugar, including no fruit, no juice, no soft drinks, and no refined carbohydrates like bread or pasta. During the three days, you can eat vegetables, plain yogurt, brown rice, and drink water. Notice if you feel better by looking at the change in your symptoms and energy level. If you do feel better, it is indicating that food is not being digested well and is producing bacterial toxins. These toxins are affecting your energy. There are many enzymes used to make energy that can become deactivated by these toxins, and therefore result in fatigue.

Lyme disease is a common, yet often hard to discover, bacterial infection that can create fibromyalgia pain. Lyme disease is a growing issue in the United States. Approximately 300,000 cases were diagnosed in 2013 according to the Center for Disease Control. The number of cases continues to grow each year as the transmission of Lyme bacteria is transmitted not just from deer ticks, but also mosquitoes. The number of cases may indeed be much higher than reported.

Lyme disease is named after the location in Lyme, Connecticut, where the disease was first identified in 1975. The local deer tick was discovered to be the transmission of the infection. In about 60 to 70% of cases, a rash may develop at the site of the bite. In 1982 the bacteria was named Borrelia burgdorferi after William Burgdorfer, Ph.D., who discovered the bacteria responsible for the infection. This Borrelia burgdorferi bacteria is corkscrew shaped that allows it to burrow and hide inside your cells. So Lyme disease is often difficult to find as the cause of a variety of symptoms. (Burrascano, 2017). The common symptoms of Lyme disease are:

➢ Fever and body aches
➢ Chronic muscle and joint pain
➢ Numbness and tingling with arm and leg weakness
➢ Bell's palsy which is paralysis of some muscles in the face
➢ Heart palpitations, shortness of breath, feeling faint
➢ Cognitive problems like memory loss and slower thinking in second stage

You can see some similarities to fibromyalgia, yet these symptoms relate to even more nervous system symptoms and excess fatigue than fibromyalgia.

Molds and Fungi

Another environmental toxin that is a growing health issue is from mold and fungi. Many serious illnesses come from mold and fungal toxicity, and there are so many types that it is often hard to find the culprit. Mold toxins are unique, and the symptoms of mold toxicity are similar to other auto-immune diseases. We have mold spores in the air, mold in foods, and mold that grows in damp environments.

Over time mold evolves into mycotoxins that cause many types of chronic symptoms. Mycotoxins feed on the nutrients in the cells where they live. They cause further weakness in the cells due to a lack of nutrients left over to help the immune system function effectively. When they cross the blood-brain barrier, they affect the central nervous system creating communication problems between nerves.

Mold spores from dead mold get inhaled into our lungs and can cause chronic coughing. Other times fungal issues show up as skin reactions. Often you can smell mold in some homes, but even when you don't smell it, it can still be there. Once I was at a seminar where we were evaluating homes that needed lots of work. One home had a noticeable mold on the walls and smelled moldy, but another house the mold was less visible but much more dangerous. I have clients move out of their home due to an unhealthy amount of mold in the house. Drier regions may still have mold problems that can be worse because the mold spores can survive in a drier climate.

Toxic molds cause increases in inflammation and show up as brain fog, memory loss, migraines, muscle cramps, tingling, insomnia, and heart palpitations. Often difficulty losing weight is another sign of potential mold issues, especially when the weight increases for no reason.

To see if you have mold in your home, I recommend using a Mold Test Kit to measure the amount of mold in your home or office. It involves putting a liquid into a petri dish and letting it sit out in a room for an hour. Then cover the petri dish and wait two days or more to see what grows in the dish. If there is growth after two days, then there is a mold problem. If there is no or very little growth after seven days, then mold may not be an issue in your environment. Mold remediation in your home can be very costly to get rid of the mold. The first step I recommend is using an air purifier that kills the fungus. Also remove any carpeting, especially if it has ever been wet.

Due to the systemic mold issues that can lurk in our body, we can do another test to see if mold is out of control in our metabolism. Do you crave sugar, or need a dessert after dinner of either a fruit or other sweet treat? You have probably heard of yeast infections which are a type of mold or fungus known as Candida.

Candida albicans is one type of systemic yeast infection that can quickly get out of control. When we overeat sugar or processed foods, are exposed to antibiotics more than once every three years, or lack sleep regularly, our immune system gets overwhelmed, and the candida yeast level gets out of control. Our gut flora controls the way we metabolize yeast and other molds. When the good bacteria in our digestive system are out of balance, this yeast will create the leaky gut environment in our intestines increasing sensitivity to regular foods. The most common signs of increased candida fungal overgrowth are new or continuing food sensitivities, stiffness and pain that are not caused by injury, unexplained, and all too often gut problems like bloating, constipation or diarrhea.

Other types of molds can get trapped in your tissues. One way to know if you might have a systemic mold is to monitor your cravings for sugar. Sugar feeds yeast or mold imbalances. To stop mold from growing in you, you will have to eliminate sugar, processed grains, like wheat, corn, rye, and barley. Also stay away from peanuts, since they grow under the ground, and often have a mycotoxin called aflatoxin. Avoid alcoholic beverages, mushrooms, and hard cheeses too.

Microwaved Food

Microwaving food is a daily convenience. Though the food still looks good, after it is cooked in the microwave oven it loses many of the beneficial phytonutrients. Using microwaves in cooking can deplete foods of their nutrients. Then when eating microwaved food, it can cause pathological changes in your body. Microwaves are high-frequency electromagnetic waves that alternate in positive and negative directions, causing vibration of food molecules up to 2.5 billion times per second. Vibrations create friction and heat, changing the chemical composition of foods and liquids. The food becomes altered so much that our digestive system has trouble breaking it down into usable nutrients.

Even water is affected by microwaves. Do you know that if you water your plants with microwaved water (after cooling it), the plants will die in just a couple weeks? It is true because the water has lost the energy to feed the plant the hydrogen and oxygen in the correct energetic configuration that correlates to the plant's needs. So do not microwave your hot water for your coffee. The loss of energy in the water will affect you too.

In an April 1992 study, the Journal of American Pediatrics reported that microwaving breast milk to warm it destroyed 98% of its immunoglobulin-A antibodies, necessary for strengthening the immune system of the infant, and 96% of enzyme activity that inhibits bacterial growth. In a German study in 1994, a comparison of the blood measurements of 8 participants who ate only traditional oven cooked foods to the blood measurement of 8 other participants who ate just microwave oven foods.

During the two-month study, blood tests were performed three times per day to measure nutrient and bacterial levels. The blood measurements of the subjects who ate the microwave food were lower in hemoglobin or red blood cells. Lowered hemoglobin can lead to anemia and thyroid imbalances. The white blood cell count increased in those who ate microwaved vegetables. This increased white blood cell count indicated that the tissues are responding to the microwaved cooked food as an infectious agent. Blood measurements also noted that the level of "bad" LDL cholesterol rose significantly after the consumption of microwaved vegetables.

While all heating methods affect the level of nutrients, microwaving foods appears to produce the most significant losses. Since we eat foods to nourish our bodies, we should daily consider what types of foods we are eating. Continuously eating foods cooked in a microwave will gradually increase the number of toxins in our systems. Eventually, the inherent healing process we all have within us will become out of balance.

Radiation, Wireless, and EMFs

A newer potential cause of chronic pain in the muscles caused by nervous system imbalances is exposure to electromagnetic frequencies. Because our nervous system has electrical impulses that create reactions we can get overwhelmed with too much electrical activity in our environment. With the increase in cell phones, wireless phones, microwaves, and modems in our home and offices we can become hypersensitive.

Often when the nervous system is already stressed, there is a higher chance to become sensitive to electrical fields. Often people don't realize they are susceptible to wireless frequencies until they make changes in their usage and exposure to their devices. I use an Electrosmog meter to measure wireless and electrical field levels in homes and offices to monitor where additional frequencies are active.

The most common symptoms of electromagnetic sensitivities are:

- ➤ Tingling or prickling sensations especially when in contact with wireless devices
- ➤ Headaches, often with nausea
- ➤ Dry mucous membranes showing up as a dry, sore throat
- ➤ Dizziness, memory loss, or lack of concentration
- ➤ Constant feeling of low-grade fever and fatigue
- ➤ Chronic aches or pains in muscles and joints
- ➤ Heart palpitations

To figure out if electromagnetic radiation frequencies are causing you pain, notice when you have these symptoms, or when they began. I have one client who has heart palpitations only when close to a modem. I have another client who had to move from an apartment that had 12 electric meters on the outside of her bedroom wall because she had severe headaches that began as soon as she moved in there.

Outside you can find out if there are antennas in your area that could be affecting your health by going to www.antennasearch.com. Cell phone towers should not be within 1000 feet of your home. Another client noticed her chronic pain and depression soon after a new tower was erected near her home. High voltage cables should also be at least 600 feet away from your home. These are known to cause immune system weakness with their constant excess emitted electrical power.

Inside your home, notice the location of your modem, Wi-Fi router, smart meters, and cordless phone charging base. All of these items emit potentially dangerous electrical fields. Also, your cell phone, especially when you initiate a call and until they answer, sends off high levels of electrical radiation. I don't recommend anyone to sleep within arm's length of their cell phone. When the wireless connection is active, there is a constant pulsing that often creates a tingling, muscle weakness, and fatigue feelings.

To see if electromagnetic frequencies are causing your fibromyalgia symptoms, do an inventory in your home and office. Find out if there is an electrical meter, any smart meters for gas, electric, or water utilities, a modem, Wi-Fi router, or cordless phone base within 6 feet of your living or working area. If so, move it, so you are not spending time close to it. I also don't recommend having any modem, mobile cell phone, or cordless phone anywhere in your bedroom, to avoid excess electrical pulsing activity during your precious sleeping time.

The electrical frequencies often have a pulse, changing from high to low constantly. These constant changing frequencies affect your nervous system as if you are struck continuously. Eventually, you will get tired of the constant irritation. If you need to use your cell phone as your alarm system, put it into airplane mode, so the wireless is off.

Chemical Toxins

Pesticides and weed killers are common environmental toxins that get into our cells and disrupt our energy. Pesticides are in and on our fruits, vegetables, and grains. Eating organic foods as much as possible is necessary to help curb the level of exposure in our daily life. Glyphosate is a chemical used in genetically engineered corn, sugar, soy and wheat products. Glyphosate kills the good bacteria in our digestive system causing many gastrointestinal disorders and increases the level of toxins that the good bacteria usually control.

Other pesticides also affect our hormone balance and raise the level of toxins in our cells that our liver has to remove. All this causes more fatigue and muscle weakness.

The digestive system needs to be functioning as effectively as possible at all times. Using herbs, acidophilus, and changing the diet are all helpful, but making sure the toxic chemicals are moved out of the organs as quickly as possible is most important. "The solution to pollution is dilution" is a phrase used to remind us to drink plenty of water every day. Keep the tissues hydrated so that toxic chemicals are flushed out before congestion occurs. One of the significant causes of constipation, skin rashes, asthma and other signs of toxin build-up is a lack of adequate water getting into the tissues. Soon we will discuss the importance of water in making sure we are hydrated enough to keep toxins out of the system and nutrients in the system.

Recommendations to Reduce Toxins

> Drink plenty of unchlorinated water, filtered to remove other toxins too, like lead and pesticides.
> Eat organic fruits and vegetables as much as possible.
> Wash fruits and vegetables with apple cider vinegar to remove any external pesticides on non-organic versions.
> Take chlorella to reduce heavy metals and EMF radiation levels.
> Take whole food antioxidant supplements to help deactivate and release toxins.
> Avoid all genetically modified foods – corn, soy, and wheat.
> Avoid food additives, MSG, high fructose corn syrup, food colorings. Read labels to make sure you are choosing clean foods.
> Do not use pesticides or weed killers in your yard. Use a white vinegar solution to kill weeds.

➢ Test for mold in your environment. There are in-home mold test kits that show if you have mold in the air.

➢ Make sure modems and wireless devices are not in your immediate environment, especially in your bedroom when sleeping.

➢ Do not eat microwaved food.

➢ Make sure your gut health is robust to fight off bacteria, viruses, and fungi.

Reducing Toxins with More Actions

What are effective ways to remove these chemical toxins from your system? First, make sure that your digestive system is working as effectively as possible. To activate the digestive juices, use fresh lemon juice in water. Lemon water will promote the proper digestion of food in the stomach.

If constipation, diarrhea, or gas and bloating are a problem, use an herbal fiber supplement. Many herbs work as cleaners or gentle laxatives to remove toxic chemicals from the colon. The most common herbal fiber supplement is psyllium husks that absorb excess wastes in the small and large intestine. Take psyllium with a good quantity of water; otherwise, the psyllium can become stuck in the colon if it is too dry for it to move through. Along with psyllium, use herbs such as cascara sagrada and senna as gentle laxatives that stimulate the muscles of the colon to move wastes through more quickly. Reduce intestinal gas with the use of peppermint or other digestive herbs. Peppermints are served in restaurants after dinner to enhance digestion so that symptoms of gas or bloating are minimized.

Another important type of herb to use to cleanse the colon is an internal moisturizer such as slippery elm or marshmallow. These herbs help keep the lining of the colon from becoming irritated. Additional herbs, such as dandelion, ginger, and yellow dock, are often included in herbal fiber cleansing to help the liver in the detoxification process. When beginning to take herbal fiber supplements, start with one-quarter of the recommended dosage, and gradually increase the dosage every few days. By steadily increasing the dosage you will prevent cleansing reactions from toxins moving out of the system too quickly.

To reduce microbes that are affecting your immune system, use homeopathic remedies designed to build up the immune system and drain toxins from the tissues. Many herbs help remove toxic bacteria and viruses. When these herbs are energized into homeopathic remedies in small doses, cleansing reactions do not cause symptoms as often, such as headaches or excessive congestion. There are drainage remedies for specific tissues and other microbial remedies that are designed to help strengthen the immune system against viruses and bacteria, including Lyme's bacteria.

Homeopathic drainage remedies help release toxins out of specific tissues. Many homeopathic remedies improve blood circulation and gently release toxins and wastes that accumulated in our muscles. Usually, detox remedies have lower potencies and are commonly used for 3 to 10 weeks depending on the level of toxicity. Drainage remedies work with detox remedies to support getting the toxins out of our organs more effectively.

The best way to effectively build your immune system is to be tested to figure out if a bacteria, virus, fungal, or chemical toxin is affecting you. A homeopathic drainage remedy supports the regeneration phase by reducing the number of toxins more efficiently.

Lifestyle

The choices we make each day create our lifestyle. How is your energy? Does it need support? Do you sleep well, or enough? Insomnia is a common symptom in the stress phase. Dietary choices are also significant in creating long term health. In this next section, we will explore all of these areas to help you understand the importance of healthy choices.

Improve Your Energy Metabolism

Do you know how your body creates energy? Mitochondria are parts of our cells that are vital to our health. Most of our cells have around 2,000 mitochondria each. To improve energy and reduce pain we need to make sure our mitochondrial can function. Our mitochondria need vital nutrients and a toxin-free environment to do their job well. Most chronic diseases from cancer to diabetes, to heart disease, and fibromyalgia are all caused by lowered energy metabolism due to weakness in the mitochondria in the cells. For fibromyalgia, the muscle cells are especially affected, so the nutrients needed for the muscles are required in higher quantities until the mitochondria are regenerated.

Mitochondria produce energy by combining the oxygen you breathe in with the food you eat. By eating foods with many antioxidants (fruits and vegetables), combined with breathing in oxygen, your mitochondria generate energy for your cells. In the process of creating energy, we produce metabolic wastes. These metabolic wastes can cause your body to age more quickly if the mitochondria are not able to release the excess wastes, or when nutrition is not available to keep the mitochondria strong.

When your metabolism malfunctions, congestion occurs in the fibrous muscle tissues due to slower circulation from lack of energy. Our bodies need energy to complete every function, from thinking, breathing, fighting illness, and digesting food, to growing new cells. The energy used by the body to do every task is called adenosine triphosphate (ATP). In most healthy cells, the mitochondria needed to create ATP are carefully maintained. But in people diagnosed with fibromyalgia, these substances may become out of balance. Adenosine triphosphate is composed of an adenosine molecule attached to three phosphate molecules. These phosphate molecules are used to help produce energy in the mitochondria energy centers of the cells, especially in the muscle and brain cells.

Research shows that fibromyalgia patients may also be deficient in certain minerals required for the synthesis of adenosine triphosphate (ATP) to create oxygen, namely magnesium and phosphorus. The energy-producing mitochondria in every cell need these minerals to produce ATP within the cells. Deficiencies slow the metabolism and increase lactic acid formation. Lactic acid causes the soreness that occurs after exercise. When this lactic acid stays in the system, this increases the amount of muscle tissue breakdown that leads to the symptoms of fatigue, depression, and muscle pain. After pain, fatigue is the second most common symptom of fibromyalgia syndrome. Studies show that both chronic fatigue syndrome and fibromyalgia may have a common link in symptoms and the metabolic factors that can cause them to occur.

Recommendations to Improve Energy Metabolism

1. Avoid eating 3 hours before going to bed. When we eat too often, especially within 3 hours before going to bed, we increase the number of free radicals that affect energy production. Since our metabolism is slower when we are sleeping, eating too close to sleeping will create excess free radicals that cause faster cell aging and mitochondrial weakness.

2. Increase your level of antioxidants daily with whole food nutrition. Eat mostly vegetables that have specific nutrients that help slow cell aging. Eat foods without a food label, like unprocessed fruits and vegetables. Or eat processed foods that have less than four ingredients, with ingredients you recognize.

3. Limit eating to just 12 hours during the day. By avoiding foods for 12 hours in the evening, your body has a better chance to use stored fat for energy. Your mitochondria can create energy from fat, and the mitochondria are more active by avoiding food for 12 hours at a time. Eating less food overall is also better for your mitochondria to stay active.

4. Take energy producing nutritional supplements. The ones I recommend most often are magnesium, B-complex vitamins, with malic acid, and an essential fatty acid combination. Get vitamins, minerals, and good fats from whole foods as much as possible. Often supplements are needed when there is a weakness in metabolism, especially if you are also diabetic.

5. Exercise and stretch daily. Stiffness and fatigue occur more when we don't move enough. Exercise also helps make your mitochondria work better. Mitochondria increase communication between your cells, and in turn, exercise helps create more energy available for your metabolism. Many people in pain avoid exercise, but regular movement and stretching are necessary to keep the energy going into the cells.

6. Reduce environmental toxins in your home. Chemical toxins in our environment affect our energy metabolism by blocking the activity of the mitochondria. Some toxins like pesticides and cleaning products weaken the mitochondria by upsetting the ability to use magnesium needed for energy in the muscles. Wireless radiation is a newer concern that causes nervous system imbalance and worsens fibromyalgia symptoms.

Get Regular Sleep

One of the most common symptoms of fibromyalgia is sleep disturbance due to chronic pain. These sleep problems can come from anxiety, which causes more muscle pain, and causes more sleep problems. Chronic pain will disrupt normal sleep cycles by acting as a stimulant, which will then affect sleeping ability even more. We need sleep to recharge our body, and when we have insomnia, we can't recharge our nervous system. Insomnia is the inability to fall asleep or stay asleep for over 2 hours at night.

Remembering the stresses of the day often causes trouble falling asleep. The body remains tense, and the adrenaline keeps flowing as long as thoughts and activities maintain stress. For at least one hour before going to bed, it is far more beneficial to engage in a quiet activity, relax in a warm bath, or meditate, than it is to watch television or do something mentally demanding. It is recommended to get between 7 and 8 hours of sleep regularly.

Sleep restores neurotransmitters. Serotonin is a neurotransmitter that fights depression and helps promote sleep. Melatonin is a hormone that enables you to sleep, by stimulating serotonin production. To restore neurotransmitters daily, it is best to get to bed by 11 p.m. Your nervous system tends to get a burst of energy between 11 p.m. and 1 a.m. if you are still awake, using more neurotransmitters to function.

For your body to operate efficiently, it must synthesize chemical energy for its various organs, cells, and processes. When your energy is low, you will be tired during the day. If you have impaired energy synthesis, you will need lots of sleep, 8 to 11 hours per day, to create energy. If you find that you feel worse during the day after less than 8 hours of sleep, this may be due to depleted energy.

Low blood sugar promotes the release of cortisone and adrenaline from the adrenals and increases liver function. If the blood sugar fluctuates during the evening, it can cause the adrenals to become more stressed, and sleep will be disturbed. Sleep disturbances are caused by many factors including the functioning of the adrenals, pancreas, and other endocrine glands. The sleep problems related to fibromyalgia syndrome are brought about by a variety of causes, and each person must look at their overall symptoms to discover how they can help themselves.

Recommendations to Help Improve Sleep:

1. Stop watching TV or using a tablet or computer for 1 hour before bedtime. Don't do any mentally stimulating work before sleeping.
2. Don't eat for 3 hours before bedtime. Your digestive system needs to be resting too to go into regeneration mode during the night.
3. Don't have your cell phone within arm's length while you are sleeping or trying to sleep. And turn off the wireless on your cell phone if it is in your bedroom. The lights and

frequencies will distract you even if you don't think you are affected.

4. Sleep in darkness. When you see light you will wake up due to changes in melatonin. To support melatonin balance, take a melatonin supplement with vitamin B6 and magnesium. This combination usually works better than plain melatonin. I recommend up to 3 mg of melatonin per day when needed. B6 and magnesium help with restless legs too.

5. A common homeopathic remedy for sleep disturbances is Coffea cruda, in a 30c potency. Yes, this remedy is made from coffee. This remedy does the opposite of drinking coffee. It won't wake you up. Take Coffea cruda when you have mental overactivity that is keeping you awake. When you are not able to turn off reoccurring thoughts blocking your sleep, this remedy is a great help. I recommend three pellets just before sleep, or as needed when you wake up during the night.

6. Use an electronic sleep tracker to see if you are sleeping soundly at night. By entering your bedtime and the time you wake up, you will find out how soundly you sleep. Then make a journal so you can track what is causing you to sleep better or worse on certain days. Is it eating later in the day or the mental stress that is keeping you awake?

7. Do you do better with a colder temperature during the night? Turn down the heat and see if you sleep better. It may take a few weeks to realize if this helps.

8. Do you need to feel pressure on your body while sleeping? Many people sleep better with extra blankets on top of them. More layers of blankets help you feel like a baby wrapped in blankets to feel more secure.

9. Another sleep technique I use successfully is to take my mind off mental stress and change focus to relaxing physically. It is called progressive relaxation. First I will tense one foot and then relax it. Progressing to the next foot – tense and

relax – until both feet are relaxed. Usually, by then, I have fallen asleep, if not I go up to my calf and then knees.

Restore Digestion

On the first day of my natural healing education, the subject was digestion. We learned, "85% of all diseases begin in the colon". As doctors of natural health, we were taught to look first for imbalances in the digestive system that could be the cause of symptoms in other parts of the body. After years of experience, I find in most cases this is true. Even when there are symptoms in other parts of the body, such as chronic upper respiratory congestion or arthritic pain, it is often initiated by imbalances in the digestive tract. The health of our whole organism is built by the foods we eat and how they digest.

The digestive process begins in the mouth. When we chew food, we break it down and digest it using the enzymes in the saliva. When the food gets to the stomach, it needs to be processed even more. The stomach needs to secrete enough hydrochloric acid to get the stomach enzymes activated. Proper secretion can take up to 30 minutes to occur. When this process takes too long, indigestion happens. When heartburn occurs, it is actually due to the lack of hydrochloric acid released on time in the stomach, which causes the food to ferment, building up gas in the stomach and esophagus, and producing pressure in the chest area.

Only by getting the stomach to secrete its hydrochloric acid and enzymes effectively will food be broken down. Taking antacids to slow or stop the secretion of hydrochloric acid inhibits the ability of the stomach to digest food properly. Antacids may help to prevent heartburn in the upper digestive tract from the mouth to the stomach, yet cause more problems in the lower digestive tract with undigested food and excess bacteria growth. Antacids also affect your ability to absorb minerals and B vitamins, especially calcium and vitamin B12.

When undigested food gets into the small intestine, it causes mucus to build up in an attempt to protect the lining of the intestinal wall. This mucus forms to counteract the bacteria created as the food ferments. The toxic bacteria flourish when food sits too long and begins to ferment or rot.In the small and large intestine, there is supposed to be a high level of good bacteria. But with fermenting food, more toxic bacteria are created. The toxic bacteria overpower the good bacteria whenever there is undigested food in the intestinal tract. If the undigested food is not removed quickly through the colon, toxic chemicals, called indicans, will form, and irritate the lining of the digestive tract.

As this irritation increases, the toxic chemicals are "leaked" through the weak cell junctions in the intestine into the circulatory and lymph system. This condition is called "leaky gut syndrome," and is linked to fibromyalgia as one of the associated syndromes. "Leaky gut syndrome" is often the cause of many chronic disease patterns. You can prevent or reverse these disease patterns by making sure you digest food in the stomach effectively by chewing very well and eating more slowly. Add probiotics to make sure you have enough good bacteria in the small intestine and colon for food to get broken down completely.

Again, the main function of our digestive system is to break down food to provide nutrients to grow, heal, and function daily. But this process can be disrupted by many factors such as the type of foods we eat, the medications we take, our exposure to environmental chemicals, and our mental and emotional stress level. These factors lead to malabsorption of nutrients caused by an imbalance of bacteria.

Malabsorption occurs when the level of mucus or imbalance of bacteria in the small intestine obstructs nutrient assimilation. SIBO (small intestine bacterial overgrowth) shows up as bloating, fullness after eating, flatulence, and either obstinate diarrhea or constipation. These same symptoms are related to irritable bowel syndrome showing that unfriendly bacteria have affected your ability to absorb nutrients. Too much toxic bacteria is the leading cause of auto-immune disorders.

The autonomic nervous system also has a third component known as the enteric nervous system located in the digestive tract. This part of the nervous system relates to irritable bowel symptoms caused by stressful activities. The enteric nervous system is affected by bacterial imbalances that modify neurotransmitters created in the small and large intestine. Mental and emotional symptoms like brain fog are often a cause of this type of neurotransmitter imbalance.

The enteric nervous system connects our brain to our gut, often called our second brain. Our emotions affect our digestive system. We may feel "butterflies" in our stomach when we are stressed. The enteric nervous system consists of over 100 million nerve cells that line our digestive tract between our esophagus and rectum. The enteric nervous system manages digestion and is essential in nutrient absorption and controlling elimination. Communication between the brain and gut affects how we think, react to foods, and our energy levels. When we are anxious, our nervous system sends signals to the gut affecting digestion ability.

Here is a complete list of symptoms of SIBO:

- Bloating and flatulence (gas) after meals
- Recurring diarrhea or constipation
- Fullness after eating
- Multiple food sensitivities

- Nausea after taking supplements
- Undigested food in stool
- Chronic sinus or urinary infections
- Muscle weakness or cramps
- Joint stiffness
- Weak or cracked nails
- Adult acne
- Iron deficiency

If you have any of these symptoms regularly, consider finding out what caused this. Common causes for imbalances of intestinal bacteria are:

- Poor diet – overeating sugar and starchy foods, food additives, and processed foods
- Eating gluten or dairy foods when sensitive to them
- Frequent antibiotic use
- Anti-acid medications used often
- A weak immune system from chronic bacterial or viral infections
- Excess emotional and mental stress
- Chronic inflammation
- Intestinal parasites that the immune system is not strong enough to ward off.

Recommendations to Improve Absorption

1. Eat unprocessed foods. Eat clean foods – no processed chemicals. Eat foods as close to nature as possible. No food labels as on whole fruits and vegetables, or labels with 4 or fewer ingredients.

2. Avoid GMO foods - Genetically modified foods cause hormonal and digestive disturbances. Corn, wheat, and soy are the most genetically modified foods, mostly to resist the accumulative effects

of pesticides. GMO foods make us more susceptible to the effects of pesticides that in turn challenge the good bacteria in our digestive tract.

3. Chew well. Most people don't chew their food enough. Carbohydrate digestion begins in the mouth. Chewing each bite at least ten times will get the digestive juices going better. Chewing can prevent the need for anti-acids.

4. Don't use anti-acids medications. They should be recommended for six months or less, but many people use them for years. Anti-acids stop the bad bacteria from being killed off in your stomach, increasing the "bad" bacterial overgrowth in your small intestine.

PH Levels and Acidity

All of the cells, organs, and fluids in your body have their ideal pH values to operate at peak performance. When the pH is higher or lower than the ideal level, your cells become stressed. Then these cells cannot use the nutrients they need, and cannot eliminate wastes efficiently until the restoration of the proper pH. Testing the pH regularly can easily monitor your pH levels.

Cell pH refers to the degree of acidity or alkalinity of the body's blood or other fluids. Calculate the number of hydrogen ions by measuring the pH levels in the blood, saliva, and urine. The term pH means "potential hydrogen," and represents a scale for the relative alkalinity or acidity of a solution. The scale begins at 0.0 with a measure of the pH of sulfuric acid and ends at 14.0 with the pH of pure calcium. The midpoint at 7.0 is a neutral reading. A reading less than 7.0 pH indicates a more acid solution, and a reading greater than 7.0 pH shows a more alkaline solution. These readings refer to how many hydrogen ions are present in the solution compared to a standard solution.

We get exposed to many types of acid and base substances that we use or consume every day. Base substances taste bitter and feel slippery or soapy. Some examples of base substances are soaps and detergents. Base substances produce hydroxyl (OH^-) ions in liquid solutions. Acid substances produce hydrogen (H^+) ions in liquids. Some examples of acid substances are citric acid found in fruits and vegetables, ascorbic acid found in fruits and vinegar, carbonic acid in soft drinks, and lactic acid found in buttermilk. Acid substances taste sour. The word "acid" comes from the Latin word *acere*, which means 'sour.' Acid liquid solutions conduct electric current, which makes them electrolytes, and react with bases to form salts and water.

Overview of pH Readings

pH	5.0 to 6.2	7.2 to 8.0
Meaning	Acid	Alkaline
Current	Increased	Decreased
Resistance	Low	High
Reactions Happen:	Too Fast	Too Slow

The pH reading is a measurement of the resistance of your tissues to electrical energy. When the pH is lower than 7.0, the current flow increases through the solution since the resistance is lower. In this case, digestive enzymes and minerals, especially calcium, move through the system too quickly to be absorbed effectively. When the pH is above 7.0, there is a decrease in the potential current flow and an increase in resistance. When the resistance increases there is less energy for the minerals and enzymes to connect, and reactions happen more slowly.

Distinct fluids have different ideal pH readings. Typically blood is slightly alkaline with readings between 7.35 and 7.45 pH. The acid/alkaline balance in the blood must be maintained daily. Calcium stored in the bone is used to keep the blood pH in balance. The pH of the urine should not get too alkaline but should stay somewhat acid. The saliva pH must not be too acid.

Optimal first morning readings after fasting all night for saliva is 6.4 to 6.8 pH, and for urine 6.0 to 6.4 pH. The urine pH reading should be lower than saliva pH in the morning since the urine is dumping residues from nighttime fasting. However, when the urine pH reading is less than 6.0 for a period of time the body begins to age more quickly, and enzymes needed to rebuild cells become inactivated. As the urine pH reading is above 6.4, it shows that the metabolism is moving more slowly, and problems such as constipation may be occurring.

Each body system has its preferred pH level that shifts during the day. Overall, the body's internal chemical environment usually changes from a weak acid to a weak base within 24 hours, generally more acid in the morning and more alkaline in the evening. The slightly acid period in the early morning is optimal for the activity of the nerves, hormones, and neurotransmitters. During the morning, the acid wastes are dissolved and eliminated in the urine.

During the day, the body buffers the pH of the food and beverages consumed by releasing electrolytes, and then the pH level goes up. This process allows the kidneys to keep the elimination process balanced. When the pH level gets too high, it indicates that the body is buffering with ammonia to compensate for a biochemical system that is too acid. Generally, when urine pH level stays below 6.0 for an extended period, it shows that the body's fluids in other areas are too acid, and it is working overtime to get rid of the excess acids.

When the urine pH is too acid, the body releases many electrolytes to keep the pH level normal and maintain life.

Two useful tests give an accurate indication of the pH of your internal environment. Use pH litmus paper to measures the pH level of the saliva and urine. The most commonly used pH papers register pH values from a moderately strong acid pH of 5.5 to a mildly alkaline pH of 8.0. The thin strip of orange-yellow paper turns color when it comes into contact with moist, or wet, acid or alkaline substances. Matching the color of the exposed litmus paper to the color on the color guide, and recording the numerical value indicated on the color guide determines the pH value. Litmus paper is most often purchased at health food stores.

The pH of your saliva can move from high to low according to what you eat during the day, and how your body metabolizes your food. To test for saliva pH, use a strip of pH test paper two inches long and create a pool of saliva on your tongue. While holding one end of the test paper, dip the other end into the saliva being careful not to touch your lips to the paper. After dipping in the saliva, immediately pull it out and read the level according to the chart. It is vital to read the paper immediately because as the paper sits in the open air, the color can change, especially if it is an alkaline reading.

Take a reading upon first rising in the morning. Ideally, the saliva pH reading should be between 6.4 and 6.8. A reading lower than 6.4 pH indicates that acid wastes are in your saliva in the morning. Test it again during the day about two hours after eating to see if the saliva pH is stable during the day. Keep a record to see the average saliva pH in the morning and during the day. If the pH value varies considerably during the day, it indicates a need to make dietary changes. It will be necessary to change the type of foods you are eating.

Salvia pH readings reflect the health of the lymph system, the upper digestive system including the stomach, pancreas and liver, and the state of the sympathetic and parasympathetic nervous system. The saliva contains an enzyme that comes directly from the liver. So the saliva pH is a good indicator of the strength of the liver. The saliva pH reveals the level of energy coming into the body. Urine pH indicates the overall function of cell metabolism, showing the level of metabolic wastes removed. When the urine and saliva pH are both acid, digestion occurs too rapidly, and more energy is used to break down tissue than to rebuild tissue. On the reverse side, when the body is too alkaline, the system moves more slowly.

Urine testing should be done upon first rising in the morning. Since the body is removing wastes overnight, the body will tend to be more acid in the morning. During the day the ideal urine pH is 6.4, but first thing in the morning it can range from 6.0 to 6.4 pH. Urine testing is best done by testing the urine in mid-stream, using either a cup to catch the urine or by using a long strip of pH paper.

The urine pH shows the level of acidity of the cell metabolism. The pH of urine can range from 4.5 to 8.0 pH. The kidneys maintain normal pH balance primarily by retaining sodium and secreting hydrogen and ammonium ions. Urine becomes increasingly acid as the amount of sodium and excess acid retained by the body increases. Alkaline urine is normally excreted when there is an excess of base or alkaline substances in the body. Secretion of acid or alkaline urine by the kidneys is one of the most important mechanisms the body uses to maintain a constant blood pH.

What exactly do low pH numbers mean? When the pH of the urine or saliva continues to be less than 6.0, the state of health becomes poor. Anxiety or chronic stress can also be affecting physiology. If mental or emotional factors are not the cause, improving diet, detoxification and gentle exercise will move the values up to the correct range. When the saliva pH is at least 6.4, it is within the healing range, which indicates that the body can come back into balance more easily with simple changes in diet. Keeping a diet diary along with your saliva and urine pH readings will show what foods are causing your body to be too acid.

Maintaining a balanced pH is essential. The pH level has a strong effect on the chemistry of our bodily fluids, either creating health or disease. Our metabolism functions more effectively with a balanced pH. Most of the regulatory processes including digestion, circulation, and breathing are altered to maintain the best pH possible. The longer the pH is out of balance, the worse the metabolism functions. Toxins will build-up more quickly and more damage will occur to our cells. The body will use acid-neutralizing minerals, such as calcium stored in the bones, to maintain a healthy balance. Poor calcium absorption is the reason we have a greater tendency toward osteoporosis as we age.

"Acidosis," is the term used to describe an imbalanced acid condition of all our body fluids. Acidosis occurs when too many hydrogen ions are measured in body fluids. Virtually all functions of the body are sensitive to the pH levels of their fluids. If the pH becomes too acid, cells become poisoned in their toxic acid wastes and die. Acidosis seriously obstructs the activities of enzymes involved in the digestive system, the nervous system and the energy operations of the body. Acidosis is caused by oxidative stress that builds up, eventually causing an increase in hydrogen ions.

Acidosis also comes from weakened oxygen metabolism in the cells and tissues. An acid pH, if left unchecked, will interrupt all cellular activities and functions, including the regularity of your heart rate and the brain function required to remember simple things. When cells are blocked by toxins or by a lack of cell flexibility, oxygen is unable to penetrate the individual cell. The cell begins to starve.

Low oxygen causes pain, fatigue, and many of the other symptoms related to fibromyalgia.

Some of the common symptoms of being too acid are tiredness, catching colds easily, pain in the muscles and connective tissues, recurring headaches, indigestion, and tightness in the chest. When the acid condition continues over a long period, excess acid substances will be created and deposited in the weakened areas of the body, so that the blood will be able to maintain its essential alkaline level. The cells around these weakened areas will either die or try to adapt to this acid environment.

The pharmaceutical companies continue to research medications to cure every type of chronic disorder. An acid/alkaline imbalance causes chronic complaints, so unless the treatment balances the cellular fluids, the 'cure' at best will be only temporary. No common drugs reduce acidity in the body. Most drugs make the body more acid. When the body extracts alkaline minerals from its cells to neutralize the acid, it causes the cells to become acid, and thus diseased. To maintain health, the majority of our diet must consist of alkaline foods.

What makes food more alkaline is the presence of organic minerals. When minerals are inherently in the food, then that food is alkaline. Foods do not become alkaline by enriching them with inorganic minerals. The Standard American Diet is high in protein, high in carbohydrate, high in fat, and is inadequate in the number of fruits and vegetables. The most commonly eaten foods are acid forming foods and will keep the body chemistry more acid. Changing the diet is the best approach to maintain appropriate pH levels throughout the body. When digested food gets metabolized, it creates either acid or alkaline pH levels in the tissues.

Protein foods such as all meats, nearly all carbohydrates, including grains, bread, pasta, and fats are acid-forming. Most fruits and vegetables are alkaline forming. Even though citrus fruits, such as oranges and grapefruit, contain organic acids and may have an acid taste, they are not acid forming when metabolized, and can make the tissues more alkaline.

To prevent cancer, the National Cancer Institute claims we need 10 to 12 servings of fruits and vegetables per day. Why is this? Fruits and vegetables are alkalizing to the system creating more oxygen in the cells. Cancer cannot live in an oxygenated environment. Daily amounts of fruits and vegetables are a dietary change that is necessary to maintain health.

Eat a diet that is 75% alkaline foods and 25% acid foods to stay healthy. The more alkaline foods we eat daily, the better we will feel. One of the fastest ways to change from an acid state to a more neutral state is to make an alkaline broth. To make this broth, combine four different alkaline vegetables, such as onions, kelp, garlic, broccoli, collard greens, and kale and simmer in water. After the vegetables have cooked and become soft, remove the vegetables and drink the broth. Drink at least one cup of broth per day, up to three cups to change a highly acid state. This broth has all the alkalizing minerals that will change the pH of the cells toward the alkaline side.

Make sure that your choice of drinks, including water, is in the neutral pH range. Soda pop is very acid with a pH between 2.0 and 3.0 pH. Coffee is also acid, as is black tea. However, green tea is an alkalizing drink and is a good choice to bring your cells back to a more neutral pH. Most types of water, with minerals still in them, are in the neutral pH range, from 6.5 to 7.5 pH. If you filter your water or drink purified water, make sure that the pH is still in the healthy range, or it will cause more stress on your cells.

There are various charts of acid and alkaline foods. Some foods begin as acids, yet when they are metabolized they create an alkaline reaction. Some examples of the foods that create an alkaline reaction but initially have an acid reaction are oranges, lemons, and apple cider vinegar. When adding sugar to any food, it makes it more acid. Also, the more processed the food, the more acid it will be, due to the preservatives in the food. The following list shows foods that tend to create acid and alkaline conditions.

Acid Creating Foods

Fruits:	Vegetables:
cranberry	peas
tomato	corn
prune	carrots
plum	Meats and Dairy Products:
dried fruits	beef
Nuts and Grains:	veal
wheat	turkey
barley	chicken
rice	ham
white bread	salmon
cashews	milk and cheese
peanuts	yogurt
walnuts	ice cream
soybeans	butter
beans	shellfish
Other:	Drinks:
sugar	coffee
chocolate	beer
honey	black tea
white vinegar	soft drinks

Alkaline Creating Foods

Fruits:

- apricots
- melons
- raspberries
- tart cherries
- mangos
- bananas
- grapes
- grapefruit
- orange
- lemon
- lime
- pineapple
- pears
- apples
- peaches
- nectarines
- watermelon
- strawberries
- tangerines
- plums

Nuts and Grains:

- almonds
- alfalfa sprouts
- oats
- quinoa
- millet

Vegetables:

- collard greens
- sweet potatoes
- potatoes
- mushrooms
- cabbage
- broccoli
- Brussels sprouts
- onions
- parsnips
- beets
- dark leafy greens
- cauliflower
- pumpkin
- sea vegetables
- kelp
- kale
- celery
- green peppers
- parsley
- squash

Drinks:

- green tea

Other:

- apple cider vinegar
- molasses

Bio-Chemical Testing for Acidosis

Saliva and urine are the most useful extra-cellular fluids used to measure the biological "terrain" which shows your overall health level. This terrain is constantly shifting depending on the demands placed on it. Every thought, feeling, and physical experience, including every stress and every bite of food eaten by you affects your biochemical systems. A variety of non-invasive saliva and urine tests measure the various chemical reactions that monitor changes in health.

One way of determining your tendency toward problems relating to imbalances in pH readings is to keep a record of your daily pH readings on the following chart. The two intersecting lines come together at a pH of 6.4, with the urine pH going vertically from 5.0 at the bottom of the chart to 8.0 at the top of the chart. The saliva pH is the horizontal line beginning at 5.0 pH on the left side and going to 8.0 pH on the right edge. By plotting your different pH readings daily, you can see in which area most of your readings are located. The more often your readings are within the square in the middle of the chart, the better your potential health level. The square contains the area of healthy first morning pH levels. The square area represents the urine pH readings between 6.0 and 6.4, and the saliva pH readings between 6.4 and 6.8.

Patterns of Stress Chart

This chart shows the four imbalances that create certain types of condition patterns.

- When both the urine and saliva pH <u>test higher than 6.4</u> there is a tendency to **toxic conditions** in the metabolism.

- When the <u>urine pH is low, and the saliva pH is high</u>, there is a tendency toward **joint and muscle stress** or pain from congestion in these tissues.
- When the <u>urine pH is high, and the saliva pH is low</u>, it can lead to **stress in the circulatory system.**
- Finally, when <u>both the urine and saliva pH are low</u> consistently, it leads to **immune stress,** where oxidative stress is causing the body to age more quickly.
- The region within the square locates the ideal urine and saliva range for first morning readings.

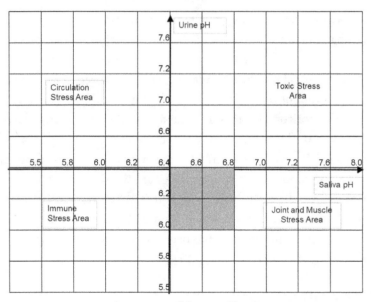

<u>Patterns of Stress Chart</u>

When both the urine and saliva pH is too high for some time, above 6.4 pH for urine, and above 6.8 pH for saliva, then the body goes into a **toxic stress** state. When this occurs, the system overloads, producing constipation and congestion. Symptoms of intestinal gas, body odors, bad breath, and a distended abdomen occur. Other symptoms related to this toxic stress state are sinus and upper respiratory congestion, skin discoloration, disk deterioration along the spine, and increased tooth decay. Alkaline pH readings indicate that the metabolism has slowed down, and there may be liver or kidney weakness.

When the saliva pH is above 6.8, and the urine is lower than 6.0, then the body goes into a **joint and muscle stress** state. The digestive system is out of balance since the upper digestive system is moving slower than the lower digestive system, creating abdominal gas and bloating. This combination creates congestion and accumulation of toxins, generating knots and lumps in the soft tissues. Fibromyalgia pain in the tender points comes from these toxins that have accumulated in the muscle tissues.

When the saliva pH is low, below 6.4, and the urine pH measures above 6.4, then there is a tendency toward a slow **circulation state**, with a movement toward having a stroke or heart attack. Also in this pattern, there is digestive stress since the upper digestive system is moving quickly and the colon area is shifting toward a slow state. Excess wastes that are created when the body is too acid are unable to move out of the system. Excess wastes cause circulation problems since the toxins created cannot be released as necessary.

When the saliva pH stays lower than 6.4 and the urine pH is lower than 6.0 for some time, the **immune system** is affected. This acid state occurs because the digestive system is moving too fast and nutrients cannot get into the cells. There will be a tendency toward fungal infections, leg cramping, and joint aching. The calcium will be drawn out of the bones to balance this acid state, so osteoporosis occurs when the body stays in this pattern. When the urine and saliva measurements regularly test with lowered pH readings, less oxygen is in the cells. This lack of oxygen in the tissues increases anaerobic bacteria and fungal growth in the body. This immune system stress will cause shortness of breath since the lungs will draw upon minerals for energy. Chronic diarrhea and other malabsorption problems will be seen, such as colitis and Crohn's disease. Also, anemia comes from prolonged acid conditions, and even supplementing vitamin B-12 and iron will not help unless pH levels are improved.

The biochemical research study results revealed that 54% of the fibromyalgia participants had saliva and urine pH results in the immune stress area, and 30% of the pH readings were in the joint and muscle stress area. Only 6% percent of the fibromyalgia group had readings in the circulatory stress area and only 2% in the toxic stress area. Just 8% of the combined saliva and urine pH readings for the fibromyalgia group were in the ideal square-shaped area.

Recommendations to Balance pH Levels

1. For at least two weeks measure your urine and saliva pH daily, upon waking up in the morning and before eating anything. You can graph your readings on the 4 section chart and see which area records most often. If your section varies from day to day, pay attention to the foods you are eating, indicating that your diet is critically affecting your metabolism.

2. Study the pH food chart in this book or download a different version at http://www.naturalchoicesforyou.com/uploads/2/5/7/0/25709329/acid_and_alkaline_chart_food_chart1.pdf

3. Do a diet diary and find out if you are eating a more acid or alkaline diet. By comparing your pH readings and foods in your diet, you can see which foods affect you exactly. Prevent many chronic diseases by keeping your pH in balance.

4. For expanded testing on pH, you can purchase and download a PDF file at: http://www.naturalchoicesforyou.com/store/p3/Are_You_Really_Healthy/pH_Testing_Kit.html This e-book has

graphs and charts that help you track your results for daily pH testing, the Patterns of Stress, the Saliva pH Challenge test with lemon, and additional tests that tell you more about your metabolism.

Oxidative Stress

The smoke we see when burning wood, or when the flesh of apples turn brown when they are cut open, are examples of oxidation in action. Oxidation, or too much oxygen, can cause the human body to degenerate, or age more quickly than usual, just as iron rusts as it breaks down. We need oxygen for life. Too much oxygen causes oxidative stress, which in turn causes chronic degenerative diseases because it, in essence, causes the human body to rust on the inside. An understanding of this oxidative process is essential to maintaining health and protecting the body from its destruction.

What causes oxidative stress? Oxidative stress appears because of too many free radicals in the tissues. Free radicals are unstable molecules looking to steal an electron from a healthy molecule. Oxygen molecules that have at least one open electron in their outer shell make up free radicals. This open electron creates an electrical charge. The free radicals attempt to get an electron from any molecule or substance in the vicinity to become stable. They move so aggressively that they chemically create bursts of light within the body. If these free radicals do not neutralize rapidly, they may produce more free radicals or cause damage to blood vessel walls, cell walls, and even the DNA of the cell. Our bodies are literally under attack potentially every minute by free radicals unless we neutralize them. Free radicals are like Pac-Man creatures that target weak areas in our body

Free radicals first attack injured or fragile tissues that did not heal well, and determine what type of diseases will develop. Some scientists believe each person has certain areas in their body that are genetically predisposed to oxidative stress, which may explain genetic-type traits when it comes to degenerative diseases. Every day in the energy center of each cell called the mitochondria; some oxidation occurs in the normal process of metabolism. Antioxidants are the best defenses against the attack of free radicals. Antioxidants bind with the extra electron in the free radical and render the free radical harmless. As long as there are adequate amounts of antioxidants in the body to handle the free radicals produced within the cell, there is no damage to the surrounding tissues.

Our daily metabolism produces many free radicals as waste products. In health, the body can neutralize and clear these chemicals. In illness, free radicals are produced in such large quantities that the body cannot neutralize them. Excess free radicals accumulate and cause oxidative stress and a buildup of metabolic toxins. The most common symptoms of metabolic toxins are digestive distress, like bloating, diarrhea, and abdominal pain. More indications of metabolic oxidative stress are shortness of breath, fatigue after eating, and obesity. Metabolic toxins become worse once oxygen metabolism becomes dysfunctional, slowing down the healing process.

Many factors increase the number of free radicals in the body. Excessive stress, excessive exercise, chemicals in our air, food, and water, cigarette smoke, microwaving foods, medications and radiation, saturated fats, and hydrogenated fats from processed foods, are all factors that increase free radicals. Margarine, made from hydrogenated fats, causes more free radicals to build up in the arteries, than butter. Butter has saturated fats, but the trans fats created from hydrogenated fats cannot be broken down by the metabolism, and live in the body as free radicals.

Stress is a fact of life, and mild or moderate stress only increases free radicals a small amount. With severe emotional stress, free radical production goes up significantly and can cause significant oxidative stress. Excessive exercise can be a cause of oxidative stress. When exercise is moderate, the production of free radicals increases, but not significantly. However, when workouts are excessive, the creation of free radicals goes up exponentially, due to lactic acid buildup. Athletes who compete regularly should be sure to get adequate levels of antioxidants regularly to compensate for their exercise regimen.

There are many more chemicals and pollutants in air, food, and water, and more people get exposed to them than ever before. These chemical toxins include pesticides, fungicides, herbicides, industrial pollutants, toxic metal compounds, and synthetic hormones. The toxic burden of chemicals has increased markedly in the last fifty years. The effects of chemical toxins show up in the body as chronic skin disorders, allergies, headaches, or lymph congestion.

Oxidative stress also comes from microbes such as yeasts, imbalanced bacteria, overactive viruses, and parasites produced even in healthy bodies. Those microbes multiply rapidly in the bowel and blood when the body has to manage other toxins from pesticides, pollutants, antibiotic overuse or sugar overload. When the level of microbes increases, the common symptoms are chronic nasal congestion, sore throat, and coughing, or chronic fatigue. All excess levels of microbes cause an increase in oxidative stress in the body that antioxidants and other nutrients have to control.

The effects of all these toxins and free radicals build up in the body causing sluggish blood flow and stagnant lymph circulation. Stiffness and pain are the most common symptoms that come from this decreased circulation. When these proteins become dense, there is a decrease in blood flow causing the congestion in the tender points. As we improve our health, we can reduce our reactions to oxidative stress.

Bio-Chemical Testing for Oxidative Stress

Biochemical tests using urine show results of oxidative stress on the body. The Free Radical Test is also called an anti-aging profile since it shows the level of stress on the body caused by free radical activity. Aging occurs more quickly when our bodies have to deal with environmental stress in the form of microbes, chemicals, and metabolic imbalances.

Free Radical Test

The Free Radical Test is a urine test that measures the level of free radical activity in the cells. When the rate of biochemical reactions in the intercellular fluid increases, there is a greater electron potential in the urine. By using a vial with malondialdehyde as the reagent, we can measure lipid peroxidation in the urine. The amount of lipid peroxidation relates to the level of tissue breakdown, which is relative to the number of free radicals in the metabolism. (Draper, 1984). The level of color change from clear to dark pink after 5 minutes is calculated.

Too many free radicals over some time lead to chronic disease and faster aging. Free radical damage comes from oxidative stress caused by heavy metals and petrochemicals in the environment and our foods, over-the-counter and prescription drugs, heated oils and fats, radiation, viruses, yeast, bacteria, and emotional stress. This test shows if you are getting enough antioxidants in your diet and supplementation program. Without adequate amounts of antioxidants, free radicals build up, and oxidative stress reactions show in this Free Radical test.

In the research project, I did free radical testing for both the fibromyalgia and control group. There are five levels of indicators of free radical levels in the test. A light pink color in the vial indicates very low free radical activity. As higher free radicals are found in the urine the color in the vial become darker pink.

Ideally, this test should be done using first morning's urine. The ideal reading is a one since everyone has some level of free radicals in their system at all times. People with fibromyalgia had an average reading between 4 and 5. You can test your level of free radicals by doing an Oxidata Free Radical stress test at home regularly to make sure you don't have too many free radicals.

Recommendations to Reduce Oxidative Stress

1. Avoid your exposure as much as possible to pesticides, herbicides, second hand smoke, cleaning solvents, and food chemicals.

2. Eat 50% of your diet as fruits and vegetables to get antioxidants in your diet.

3. Take whole food antioxidant supplements to increase your amount of plant nutrients in your cells. Read the next section to learn more specifics.

4. Order a free radical test kit to test your level of free radicals to make sure you are getting enough antioxidants. Get Oxidata free radical test kits at www.naturalchoicesforyou.com

Antioxidants and Free Radicals

Decreasing our exposure to risk factors that create free radicals is just the beginning of staying healthy. We can't eliminate all free radicals without the support of antioxidants. There must be enough antioxidants to handle all of the free radicals produced, or oxidative stress will create degenerative diseases. Free radicals inflict some damage to our cells, even when we have adequate antioxidants. However, our body has a great ability to heal itself with the proper nutrients.

When there is a lot of stress or acidity in the system, free radicals will thrive. The excess free radical activity comes from an impaired metabolism or an immune system response to environmental toxins or allergens. Free radicals are highly reactive chemical ions. They cause microscopic tissue damage to body proteins producing hardening in the soft tissues. Increasing dietary antioxidants along with minerals will reduce free radicals. The body can make some antioxidants. Two of them are called superoxide dismutase (SOD) and catalase. However, the body is not able to produce enough of these antioxidants on its own to neutralize all of the free radicals that are present. Adequate amounts of antioxidants need to be supplied daily through our food and the use of supplements. The most common vitamin antioxidants are vitamins A, C, and E.

Vitamin C is water-soluble and the most effective antioxidant for the health of the blood. Vitamin C is essential for the strength of the connective tissue, and the support of bones, blood vessels, joints, organs, muscles, eyes, teeth, and skin. Vitamin C helps with antibody production and white blood cell activity. It can help reduce cholesterol and protects your heart. Since it is water-soluble, it protects the watery tissues of your body including your sinuses. Vitamin C also helps to manufacture neurotransmitters like serotonin and dopamine, protects the gall bladder from gallstones, and improves the transport of iron into cells.

Vitamin E is a fat-soluble vitamin and the most effective antioxidant for the health of the cell wall. Vitamin E is found in four vital tocopherols compounds called alpha-tocopherols, beta-tocopherols, gamma-tocopherols, and delta tocopherols. The most common form of Vitamin E in supplements is alpha-tocopherol. All of the tocopherols are found in whole vegetables and work together to support the immune and circulatory systems. Vitamin E destroys free radicals, helps to heal the skin, fights disease and helps reduce heart problems. Also, vitamin E is beneficial in reversing calcium build-up in the soft tissue and easing stiffness in the connective tissue. When consumed together, Vitamin C improves the effectiveness of vitamin E and may block some of the harmful effects of a high-fat meal.

Make sure when you have a supplement with vitamin E that it is the natural form. The common synthetic form of vitamin E is listed as **dl**-alpha-tocopherol. The natural form will not have the "l" after the "d," and will read as **d**-alpha-tocopherol. Many studies show that synthetic vitamin E does not have the same protective qualities as natural alpha-tocopherol. Ideally, get a full complement of vitamin E with all four compounds.

Vitamin A is another fat-soluble nutrient stored in the liver. It comes into the body from beta-carotene, one of the twenty-two carotenoids found in fruits and vegetables. Vitamin A is needed for the health of the immune system and helps with reproduction of cells in the respiratory and digestive tract. It is also necessary for good night vision and helps to prevent dry eyes. Supporting eye health is why our mothers told us to eat carrots. The orange color in the carrot is full of carotenoids and therefore helps with many aspects of our vision. By combining vitamin A with all the other antioxidant vitamins, the metabolic process will be more efficient, excess free radicals will decrease, energy levels will improve, and pain will subside. There must always be an abundant supply of antioxidants within every cell and tissue to protect the body against free radicals.

In addition to these vitamins, there are thousands of other antioxidants obtained from foods, primarily fruits, and vegetables. **Phytochemicals**, or plant chemicals that have the toughest antioxidant properties, are found in fruits and vegetables. The various colors reveal the benefit of fruits and vegetables. Deeper colors indicate a superior amount of phytochemicals. Red foods help strengthen the blood. Green foods have the whole vitamin E compound and benefit the circulatory system. Orange colored foods have many antioxidants including vitamins A and C. There are more than one thousand types of phytochemicals. An apple has more than 300 different phytochemicals that improve our health when we eat the apple. The higher the varieties of phytochemicals in the diet, the better the chance for free radicals to be reduced.

There is no way each of the phytochemicals can be broken down effectively into separate supplements. It is best to get them from the daily diet or whole food supplements. Alpha lipoic acid, mixed carotenoids, ubiquinol, indoles, N-acetyl-cysteine, lutein, and bioflavonoids are examples of identified phytochemicals, available in whole foods to help us in the battle against free radicals. Sulfurophane is a phytochemical found in broccoli that helps to shrink cancerous tumors. But sulfurophane does not work well unless combined with all of the other phytochemicals in the broccoli. Not only do these phytochemicals and antioxidants work in synergy with one another, but also they work against different types of free radicals.

How many antioxidants do you need? Vitamins A, C, and E are better metabolized and absorbed into the system when supplied together in foods, than when taken separately. The commonly recommended dosage of vitamin A is 5000 I.U., vitamin C is 500 mg, and vitamin E is 400 I.U. per day. More antioxidants are needed when eating the standard American diet that contains too many synthetic chemicals and hydrogenated oils found in most processed foods. The partially hydrogenated fats are not broken down in the system and create many free radicals. Excessive cholesterol is formed to protect the arteries from the free radicals that are produced from eating these fats. Individuals need to take higher doses of antioxidants with these fatty meals so that these effects can be eliminated. Also, if you have a tendency to sinus congestion, or have a susceptibility to colds and other viruses, then you will need additional antioxidants.

Antioxidants by themselves are not the complete answer. They work more efficiently with adequate amounts of minerals, including trace minerals such as copper, zinc, manganese, and selenium. Also, there must be sufficient amounts of B complex vitamins to support the enzymatic reactions of the antioxidants. If these minerals and B complex vitamins are not present in adequate amounts, even when antioxidants are present, oxidative stress will still occur.

The American Cancer Society recommends that we each eat 9 to 13 servings of fruits and vegetables daily. Only 10% of the United States population gets the minimum of five servings per day. The fruits and vegetables should be in a variety of colors to be the most beneficial. Vegetables such as kale, parsley, spinach, broccoli, and beets are very dark in color, which indicates that they are more nutritious. Taking supplements made from whole food sources helps the body maintain a consistent amount of strong antioxidants, minerals, and enzymes in the digestive system that helps to fight free radicals.

When taking antioxidant food supplements, your body will gradually improve its metabolism. Food supplements need to be consumed for at least three months to recognize their effectiveness. The effects will be cumulative. As the nutrients build up in your system, you will begin to feel the difference enhanced nutrition makes.

Use Minerals to Increase Cell Energy

To make the energy we need daily, we need to have a balance of minerals. Each mineral depends on other minerals to work effectively. Minerals are also known as co-enzymes, working with enzymes to help create energy in the growth and function of the tissue. Minerals specifically help form bones and the blood, keep the nervous system functioning, and regulate the activity of the muscles. There are two types of minerals, macrominerals and trace minerals. The macrominerals are required in larger amounts than the trace minerals. The macro minerals are calcium, magnesium, potassium, sodium, and phosphorus. There are many trace minerals, but the most common are zinc, copper, iron, silicon, manganese, sulfur, chromium, iodine, and selenium. It is possible to create mineral toxicity from taking too many minerals. However, to accumulate too many minerals, they would have to be overly consumed, in inorganic form regularly, for an extended period.

Calcium

Calcium is the most abundant mineral found in the body. It is found mostly in the bones and teeth, and the rest is in the soft tissues. Calcium is needed for muscles to contract, and to regulate the nervous system. Calcium determines the volume and density of each cell, affects the cell's ability to absorb nutrients, and controls the metabolic acids. When there is a calcium deficiency, the muscles cannot efficiently absorb any of the minerals they need. Calcium is needed more than any other mineral; yet, it is best absorbed from whole plants instead of with inorganic supplementation. Calcium is found in almonds, egg yolks, dark leafy green vegetables like kale, spinach, cabbage, and in most dairy products. Sugar in the daily diet depletes calcium since it increases acidity, which requires the use of more calcium to maintain balance.

In fibromyalgia, calcium is especially needed to balance the acid/alkaline levels and to reduce stress in the muscle and nervous system. The liver needs sufficient amounts of calcium; otherwise, the metabolism of the whole body is affected. There are many types of calcium available on the market. When the urine pH level is too low, under 5.5, calcium carbonate can be absorbed. At pH levels between 5.5 and 6.2, calcium citrate is absorbed well. When the urine pH readings are higher than 6.4, calcium lactate is better absorbed. Vitamin D3 is especially needed to absorb calcium when the pH is too low. The lower the urine pH, the more vitamin D3 is needed to help calcium be absorbed.

The amount of calcium needed per day is dependent on the type of calcium used, and how well it will be absorbed. Calcium needs magnesium, zinc, phosphorus, silica, and boron along with vitamin D3 to be absorbed effectively. Excess calcium that is not absorbed builds up in the tissues of the joints and arteries, which makes it very important not to take too much calcium.

Magnesium

For fibromyalgia pain, **magnesium** is the primary mineral needed to reduce stress in the muscles. Magnesium is the fourth most abundant mineral in the body, and the second most abundant in the muscle tissue, after potassium. Magnesium helps to relax muscles, expand airways, and regulate heart rhythms. Magnesium is needed for over 300 enzyme reactions and is the major mineral required for energy formation. Deficiencies of magnesium can cause swelling of the cell membranes, hardening of the soft tissues, sleep disturbances, and irritability.

Magnesium is one of the most crucial elements for the production of adenosine triphosphate (ATP). The entire energy production system is dependent on magnesium, and even a slight magnesium deficiency can slow down the production of ATP. Oxygen deficiency in the cells can come from a lack of magnesium available to the energy cells, or mitochondria. Without the proper amount of oxygen and magnesium, lactic acid builds up causing soreness, lung capacity decreases causing shortness of breath, and fatigue increases.

Research shows that most fibromyalgia patients have below-normal levels of magnesium. Low levels of magnesium contribute to many common complaints. Here is a list of symptoms common to magnesium deficiency:

- Muscle cramps or spasms
- Chronic pain
- Headaches or migraines
- Chronic fatigue
- Poor sleep
- Numbness and tingling in the extremities
- Restless legs
- Eye twitching
- High blood pressure, heart palpitations, abnormal heart rhythms
- Acid reflux
- Constipation
- Sensitivity to loud noises
- Anxious, irritable, or depressed
- A feeling of overwhelm or uncontrollable stress
- Recurring bacterial, viral, or fungal infections
- Fasting blood sugar above 100

From this list, you may realize that magnesium deficiency may be a predictor of future diabetes and heart disease because the symptoms are similar to diabetes and heart issues. Adding magnesium to your diet daily can reduce your risk and reverse the damage caused by the lack of this necessary nutrient.

Many common foods Americans eat do not contain enough magnesium. Magnesium is found in whole grains, dark green leafy vegetables, kelp, and many kinds of nuts and legumes. At least 85 percent of magnesium is removed from bleached and refined flour in bread, pasta, and other prepared wheat products. Poor diet also contributes to magnesium deficiency. Here are common dietary causes that lead to low magnesium in the tissues:

- Eating sweets regularly
- Drinking more than two soft drinks per week
- Drinking coffee or other caffeinated drinks daily
- Regular strenuous exercise
- Taking a diuretic, heart medication, asthma medication, or birth control pills
- Taking calcium supplements without equal parts of magnesium

Any type of refined sugar in our diets will cause our body to excrete extra magnesium through the kidneys. Sugar has no nutrition. When we eat more sugar, the more minerals and B complex vitamins we need to metabolize that sugar.

Dark colored soft drinks have phosphoric acid that affects bone strength by binding with calcium and magnesium and making them unavailable to make energy and build healthy new tissues. Consumption of soft drinks has dramatically increased in the past 20 years along with the increase in chronic disease patterns like fibromyalgia and diabetes. I have a friend that needed hip replacement surgery in her 40's because she drank Coke as her beverage of choice. Her hip bones became weak to the point they essentially disintegrated, and she had no strength.

Uncontrolled stress can be a cause of magnesium deficiency. But also a lack of magnesium tends to magnify the sensation of stress in our lives. When we feel "stressed," with a feeling of overwhelming anxiety, look at a need for magnesium. Our adrenals need minerals, especially magnesium to react effectively to stressful events.

Eating foods rich in magnesium throughout the day is the best way to get this mineral absorbed into your system. The best source of magnesium in your diet is from green vegetables. The dark green color comes from the chlorophyll which contains magnesium. Spinach, kale, collard greens, and dark lettuces have magnesium. Also, unprocessed whole grains, like wheat bran and whole oats, along with nuts contain magnesium. Here is a list of foods and the amount of magnesium in a single serving:

Food	Milligrams of Magnesium
Wheat bran, ¼ cup	89
Almonds, roasted, 1 ounce	80
Spinach, cooked, ½ cup	78
Raisin bran cereal, 1 cup	77
Cashews, roasted, 1 ounce	74
Soybeans, cooked, ½ cup	74
Wheat germ, ¼ cup	69
Oatmeal, cooked, 1 cup	61

Calcium and magnesium work together for proper metabolism. A few years ago the recommended calcium to magnesium ratio was 2:1. Now the ratio has shifted to an equal amount due to the levels of daily stress reactions we have. An excess of calcium in the system will deplete magnesium levels. Magnesium is a common deficiency with those who have a high dairy intake. Milk has a calcium/magnesium ratio of approximately 10 to 1, which tends to decrease magnesium levels. Excess consumption of calcium, refined carbohydrates, alcohol, or fats can deplete magnesium.

Our body only absorbs about 50% of magnesium in our foods and supplements. And 75% of people in the US take in less than the RDA. How much magnesium do we need daily? The recommended daily requirement of magnesium is 320mg for adult women and

420mg for adult men. The average amount consumed in the United States is about 1/2 that amount.

For fibromyalgia pain relief, I recommend a minimum of 400mg of magnesium per day. It may be necessary to begin with up to 800 mg per day of magnesium citrate, magnesium aspartate, or magnesium glycinate. If you tend towards loose bowel function, don't use magnesium citrate due to its laxative quality. Magnesium aspartate is absorbed better in the muscles to enhance athletic performance.

Magnesium also helps reduce the stress to our nervous system from EMF radiation in all of our wireless technology. Aluminum toxicity may also play a role in symptoms experienced by people deficient in magnesium, so magnesium supplementation can help block the toxic effects of aluminum. However, the most potent aluminum detoxifier is malic acid. Malic acid is especially effective at decreasing aluminum toxicity in the brain. Clinical tests show malic acid to be a great asset in the treatment of fibromyalgia pain especially when in combination with magnesium.

Malic acid in supplementation with magnesium improves the amount of oxygen and energy available to the cells. Malic acid is found in many citrus fruits and apples. The Journal of Nutritional Medicine published a study on the combined effects of magnesium and malic acid for fibromyalgia clients. Their test used 1,200 to 2,400 mg of malic acid with 300 to 600 mg of magnesium for 4 to 8 weeks with 15 clients. The results of their study showed a significant amount of pain relief within 48 hours, and a measurable decrease in pain in the tender points. (Abraham, 1992;3)

Malic acid helps reverse muscle weakness by getting more oxygen to your cells. Malic acid is found in food but also is made during the Kreb's energy cycle. By supplementing malic acid more oxygen becomes available in the cells and more energy can be created helping specifically to improve physical exertion levels. Malic acid helps open up blocked energy production in the mitochondria. Often malic acid is combined with magnesium in supplements made explicitly for fibromyalgia.

The need for **potassium** is increased if too much magnesium is consumed at once. Potassium deficiency can cause severe muscle cramps, restlessness, and irregular heartbeats. Cramps are quickly reduced with the use of 100-200 mg of potassium in tablet form. Fruit and vegetable juices contain 200-500 mg of potassium per cup, depending on the type of fruit or vegetables used. A whole banana contains around 390 mg. of potassium. A high amount of potassium is also found in oranges, potato skins, and kelp. Potassium is depleted by sweating, or by using diuretic substances such as medications or caffeine.

Sodium must be kept in balance with potassium. Sodium retains fluids, while potassium is a diuretic. Organic sodium is found in many fruits and vegetables especially celery and kelp. Organic sodium is not the same as table salt or inorganic sodium chloride. Both organic sodium and potassium are essential for proper nerve function, especially of the heart. An imbalance of organic sodium and potassium can cause nerve symptoms such as muscle discomfort, restlessness, twitching, and chronic fatigue. Additionally, potassium is not stored in the tissues without adequate magnesium. So all four minerals: calcium, magnesium, sodium, and potassium, must be in balance as a group. An excess of any one of them may do as much if not more damage than a deficiency.

Trace minerals assist in the absorption of the macrominerals. For example, calcium is absorbed well when combined with magnesium, phosphorus, and trace minerals manganese, silica, boron, and zinc. Manganese helps carry oxygen throughout the body and strengthens the connective tissues. It is a mineral found in whole grains, nuts, and egg yolks. Iron is a component of red blood cells and helps get oxygen into the blood and muscles. Iron is found in beef liver, kelp, and molasses. Silica is a mineral that aids in strengthening nails, hair, and teeth. It is a trace mineral that is important for the brain and nervous system and is found in green leafy vegetables, apples, almonds, and sunflower seeds. Zinc is another trace mineral that is needed by the immune system. It helps in wound healing, the formation of DNA and protein, and improves hormonal function. Zinc is found in sunflower seeds and nuts.

B-complex vitamins are vital nutrients to help minerals support the nervous system, control anemia, help with memory, and relieve dizziness, headaches, and insomnia. B complex vitamins are found in many nuts, legumes, and protein foods, like meat and dairy foods. When using supplements, it is best to use B-vitamins in a complex, or combined form. They are absorbed more efficiently when taken together.

There are some common foods that contain many minerals. Garlic is one of those foods. Garlic has many minerals and phytochemicals. That is why it helps improve the functioning of the immune system and is known as the poor man's antibiotic. Kelp is a type of seaweed that contains many types of minerals. Dark green vegetables have many antioxidants, all of the macro minerals and many of the trace minerals. Eating a salad with a variety of vegetables a day will help you get the full complement of the major minerals you need each day.

Essential Fatty Acids and Cell Nutrition

If you have dry skin, stiffness, concentration problems, or hormonal imbalances you may be lacking in a type of fat that is essential to health. Essential fatty acids (EFA) are those fats that the body needs, yet it cannot synthesize itself. Fatty acids are the building blocks of our cell membranes. Although many types of fat are unhealthy fats, some are beneficial and necessary. Cutting all fat from the diet is harmful to health.

Do you lack essential fatty acids? Here are common symptoms related to low EFAs:

➢ Joints are achy or stiff
➢ Skin is dry or flaking
➢ Nails are soft or brittle
➢ Thirsty often
➢ High blood pressure
➢ High cholesterol

Essential fatty acids are critical in the proper metabolism of fats. The standard American diet mainly consists of fats that are deficient in these essential nutrients. Partially hydrogenated oils that are found in snack foods are detrimental to health. These types of fats, found in most vegetable oils, are converted to trans-fatty acids when heated, or oxidized. This is the type of fat that increases cholesterol in the arteries. These trans-fatty acids can't be used by the body and link to many severe health conditions, such as heart disease and cancer. Saturated fats are another type of fat found in red meats and dairy foods.

Essential fatty acids are essential in many metabolic processes, including energy production. Since the body cannot produce them, they must be consumed in the diet to optimize health. The essential fatty acids are the omega-3 (linoleic) and omega-6 (linolenic) fatty acids. These nutrients are the main structural components of the body's cell membranes, are crucial to optimum performance, and can enhance overall health if they are present in adequate quantities.

Omega-3 and omega-6 are also vital in preventing damage from other fats.

One of the reasons to take essential fats is to balance prostaglandins. Prostaglandins act on specific areas of injury in the body by attaching to cell receptors. Prostaglandins act as signals to control healing in the area of the body where they are made. They create fever, pain, and inflammation to begin the healing process. Different prostaglandins stimulate or suppress actions needed in healing. Prostaglandins also regulate the contraction and relaxation of the muscles in the lungs and gut. Prostaglandins do their specific action and then are broken down, so they do not stay in the body to work in other areas.

High levels of prostaglandins are made when you are injured or have an infection. Chronic inflammation occurs when the tissues continue to request or need high levels of prostaglandins due to poor healing ability.

Omega-3 and omega-6 are the two polyunsaturated fatty acids that are necessary to produce prostaglandins to regulate many functions in every cell of the body and to produce energy. Prostaglandins increase the metabolic rate and stamina and decrease recovery time from fatigue. These fatty acids help to form the structural part of all cell membranes, regulate the flow of substances into and out of the cells, and protect the cells from invading bacteria, viruses, allergens, and other toxins. Essential fatty acids are especially needed for proper brain functioning.

Every cell in the body is like a tiny factory, taking in raw materials from the surrounding fluid and sending out various chemicals. Everything going into or coming out of the cell has to pass through the cell's membrane. The membrane depends on essential fatty acids to remain fluid and flexible. Without them, the membrane becomes stiff and unable to do its job.

Essential fatty acids are also imperative in oxygen transfer and red blood cell production. They shorten recovery time from fatigue since they encourage the blood to bring vital oxygen to muscle cells and they enable the cells to more easily absorb nutrients needed for recuperation.

The benefits realized by regular use of essential fatty acids:

- Improved cholesterol levels
- Lower blood pressure
- Improved memory
- Increased circulation
- Reduced joint stiffness
- Reduced dryness of the skin
- Enhanced immune system function
- Less inflammation
- Balanced hormones
- Better moods.

As you can see, fatty acids are essential for metabolism and health. Flax oil is the richest vegetarian source of omega-3 fats. Flax oil can be used in salads in place of other salad dressings. Flax oil shouldn't be used for cooking, as high heat damages the fatty acids. Other sources of omega-3 fatty acids are fish oils from salmon, tuna, and cod.

Omega-6 fatty acids are found in many cooking oils such as vegetable oils of soy, corn, and sunflower oil. These are not beneficial omega-6 oils because of how they break down in our metabolism. Better omega-6 oils are borage and evening primrose oil. These omega-6 acids are the precursors of gamma-linolenic acid (GLA). Supplements providing GLA, such as primrose oil, helps the body make prostaglandins, the substances that help to relax muscles that tend to cramp.

Both omega-3 and omega-6 fatty acids are supplements to be added in the diet. The ideal ratio of these fats for healthy people is two parts omega-6 to one part omega-3. Since more omega-6 is eaten in the common diet of Americans, this ratio is often out of balance by as much as 6:1. For people who have immune system weakness, heart disease, blood sugar imbalance, and fibromyalgia, there is a need to increase the amount of omega-3 fats so that the prostaglandins can get into a better balance. Increasing the number of fish oils and flax oil will help especially get the omega-3 fatty acids into the metabolism. A 2000 mg quantity of flax oil is usually equivalent to 2 capsules or 1 tablespoon and is the recommended minimum per day.

The omega-3 and omega-6 fats need catalysts to be absorbed in the body. These catalysts are vitamins B3 (niacin) and B6, vitamin C, and the minerals magnesium and zinc. When these nutrients are not sufficient, then the essential fatty acids will not be absorbed well. Also, when too many partially hydrogenated oils or trans fats are part of the standard diet, then supplementation of essential fatty acids is less effective.

The omega-3 fatty acids have a beneficial blood thinning effect that enables more blood to reach the muscle cells. More blood means more oxygen is available to those muscles, which will lead to reduced recovery time and less pain.

Other positive health effects of essential fatty acids are enhanced anti-oxidant activity, cardiovascular protection, healthy skin, anti-microbial activity, and tumor inhibition. Their primary role in a healthy body, however, is in energy production. When added to the diet, they are alkalizing to the system. Similar to most nutrients, essential fatty acids are best supplied with the other essential nutrients that our body requires.

A combination of essential fatty acids, minerals, enzymes, and antioxidants, are all needed to make the metabolic changes that reverse fibromyalgia symptoms. By looking at the imbalances in each area of metabolism and the recurring symptoms, the necessary need for each type of supplement can be decided.

Recommendations to Balance Antioxidants, Minerals, and Essential Fatty Acids:

1. Take a high-quality whole food antioxidant supplement. I do not believe we can get all the nutrients we need from our diet due to inadequate soil nutrients. I recommend taking a whole food antioxidant or multi vitamin and mineral supplement.

2. Get extra minerals, especially magnesium. I recommend at least 400 mg of magnesium, up to 800 mg per day. Don't buy magnesium oxide; it is not absorbed well. Get either magnesium citrate, or glycinate, or aspartate. These forms of magnesium are easily absorbed. If you take too much magnesium citrate, you may get diarrhea effects.

3. Along with the magnesium, add malic acid to increase the amount of oxygen that gets into the cells to created energy. Many fibromyalgia supplements combine magnesium with malic acid and specific B vitamins to help reduce pain effectively.

4. Take a B-complex vitamin supplement with the magnesium to increase the action of both supplements. I especially recommend getting enough B1 (thiamine), B6, and B12 for increased energy metabolism.

5. Take a minimum of 2000 mg of essential fatty acids daily. Take fish oils to increase flexibility and energy production in the cells. You may need up to 4000 milligrams or even more at first to energize

the metabolism. Add evening primrose oil to help with stiffness and when you have hormone imbalances. Usually, I recommend twice as much omega-3 oils (fish or flax oil) as omega-6 oils (evening primrose oil or borage oil.) Avoid soybean oil, corn oil, and all partially hydrogenated oils.

6. Work up gradually the number of supplements until you get relief of stiffness and pain. I usually recommend increasing the amount of each supplement every five days if you do not see a result you expect. With the best balance for your needs, you will see a significant improvement in your health.

The Importance of Water

Water in our cells is vital. Our blood contains about 55% plasma, and the plasma is about 92% water. That makes our blood just less than 80% water. Overall, our body has about 64% water weight, unless we are dehydrated. Dehydration happens when we don't drink enough water to replace water loss through urination, breathing, and sweating. Hydration is essential to release toxins we accumulate daily.

When you have pain in a specific area, it is because the energy of the fluid in those tissues is not flowing smoothly. Can you feel this lack of flow in your tissues? I have clients that recognize precisely where the water is not flowing. Being aware of water energy in your tissue helps you decide which tissues to focus on for healing. If you don't take in an adequate amount of water, you will be more prone to chronic disorders like obesity, constipation, nausea, headaches, asthma, arthritis, and of course, fibromyalgia. Unfortunately, not many people drink as much water as they need.

Are you dehydrated? It is not easy to tell. There are different types of devices to monitor skin hydration and internal hydration. Some body composition scales measure hydration and can give you an idea of how well you are absorbing the water you are drinking. Bioelectrical impedance analysis (BIA) is another test to show you the amount of water in your body. BIA uses a mild electrical current that travels between electrodes on the body to measure the resistance of the flow. BIA is commonly used by weight loss nutritionists to help measure the amount of fat, muscle, and other metabolic factors affecting weight.

There are symptoms you can monitor to see if you are dehydrated. One is the color of your urine when you wake up in the morning. Darker urine color indicates that it is more concentrated. It should be a slight yellow color in the morning, not clear, but also not dark yellow or brownish. Do you wake up thirsty? Thirst can be an indication that you need to drink more water during the day.

A common recommendation is to get one-half your weight in ounces per day of water. For example, if you weigh 150 pounds, you would need to drink 75 ounces of water (only counting pure water) per day. This amount of water may be too little or too much for some people. The type of water you are drinking can determine if it is staying in your cells or just passing through your kidneys. Only one-half of the fluids in coffee, tea, wine, or soft drinks count towards your daily water amount.

Water inside cells is called the interstitium. Interstitial fluid increases during inflammation showing up as swelling or edema. Water in our cells holds memories and is active in our body's intelligence activity. Remember from the 5 phases of the healing process that our organ tissues direct the regeneration process after experiencing stressful events or repeating patterns. The intelligence of our body helps specific brain areas direct the healing phases. When we have symptoms, we need to deal with the physical symptoms, yet we also have to consider the message that our intelligence is trying to tell us. Does a pain symptom show up to make us aware, so we don't repeat the same pattern again? Remember that symptoms are our body's way to restore order to correct a stressful event.

Fluid in cells communicates information by imprinting energy patterns. Since all blood flows through the heart, the fluid in the blood affects our emotions and memories that we feel. Do you have repeating patterns or habits in your life you want to change? Often these patterns show up to let us know we are not learning what we need to learn. Water wants to flow easily, and does that better when it is pure, containing positive emotions instead of negative habit patterns. Positive emotions such as love and gratitude make our hearts more joyful, reducing feeling overwhelmed and anxious.

You can ask questions to help figure out why water is getting congested in your tissues. Why is the fluid not flowing? Did something happen to cause this? Is there something for you to learn from this congestion pain? What energy is needed to solve this problem? An awareness of these answers will improve your water flow energy.

<u>What Type of Water is Best?</u>

There are many types of water for you to choose to drink. My first choice is to find water without chlorine. The amount of chlorine in most city tap water varies from day to day. To discover the level of chlorine in tap water, use a pool chemical test kit and look at the chlorine level. Very often the amount of chlorine found in tap water is so high that it is at an unacceptable swimming level, and is dangerous to drink or shower in regularly.

Carbon filtering takes many of the inorganic minerals, like chlorine, out of the water. It is one of the most common ways of making tap water safe to drink. Reverse osmosis water filters out most of the chemicals and bacteria, flushing the wastes out with the excess water that is discharged. This water is pure, as is steam-distilled water, which also has all the inorganic minerals removed. I use a counter top reverse osmosis water system for my drinking water at home. I do add trace minerals to my water daily to compensate for the lack of minerals.

Bottled water comes in a variety of forms. Some choices are spring water that comes from a natural spring; others are carbon-filtered tap water, reverse osmosis filtered water and steam distilled water. Bottled water has many different potential qualities. Unless you know exactly the form of the water that you are buying and have it tested for chlorine and pH, you may not know what you are drinking.

There is a controversy about which type of water is better. Purified water has less than 10ppm of impurities, which is better than spring water. Spring water has more minerals, so it can stick to your cells better providing better hydration. Ideally, you can add trace minerals, or Himalayan pink salt or Celtic sea salt to your purified water so that it has minerals in it. It also makes it have a more satisfying taste. You will notice that you are not urinating as often when you have minerals added to your water, helping with hydration. You can measure the pH of your water to see if it has minerals in it. If the pH is lower than 6.2, it doesn't have enough minerals.

Drinking more water can eliminate excess fat. Your body uses water to transport nutrients into your blood and to take wastes out of your system. A lack of water in the tissues causes toxins and fats that are typically discharged, to remain in your tissues. That extra weight you think of as fat may not be fat at all. It may be fluid retention that exists to protect you from toxins that have built-up in your connective tissues. Spreading out the amount of water throughout the day is more comfortable on your kidneys and helps to control body chemistry better in the liver. Drink only 8 to 12 ounces at a time. Drinking too much water, over 16 ounces at one time, too often, will stress the kidneys.

<u>Lemon Water</u>

The liver needs proper hydration to keep oxygen balance in the brain for nervous system messaging. Adding fresh lemon juice to your water every morning can strengthen your liver and improve your natural detoxifying ability. Add one tablespoon of freshly squeezed lemon juice to 8 ounces of water in the morning to help activate the digestive enzymes in the liver, and regulate the amount of oxygen in the blood. Frozen or concentrated lemon juice is processed and does not contain the enzymes needed to support the liver.

Fresh lemon juice contains citric acid, which is the primary carrier of biochemicals in the body's energy system. Lemon juice has been known to cleanse the kidneys of small calcium stones by breaking down calcium deposits. If the kidneys are too stressed, causing middle back pain or frequent or burning urination, then lemon juice is not recommended. Or if you are too low in magnesium or potassium, lemon juice is not recommended. If the lemon juice is tolerated well, it is recommended to take it regularly two to three times during the day. Lemon water will strengthen the liver and help to balance the biochemistry of the tissues.

<u>What about Soft Drinks?</u>

Soft drinks, or carbonated drinks, are the beverage of choice in America for many people. Drinking this flavored carbonated water with preservatives could be one of the most harmful habits we have. Added sugar and phosphoric or citric acid increase the acidity of the drink. Soft drinks have a pH level between 2.0 and 3.0 pH, compared to water that has a pH between 6.6 and 7.4. Constant consumption of acid beverages increases the acidity in the tissues that can lead to anemia and nervous system weakness.

Sweeteners, such as high fructose corn syrup and aspartame, are other components of soft drinks that make them more acid. One 12-ounce can contains 7 to 10 teaspoons of high fructose corn syrup. Excessive fructose in the diet leads to stress on the liver and immune system, weakening of teeth, and excess depletion of vitamins and minerals received from the healthy foods. Fructose causes fermentation in the digestive system, affecting beneficial bacterial growth and altering the absorption of nutrients. In the digestive process, excess fructose stops the liver from working with the pancreas to keep the blood sugar in balance. Now many people know the dangers of high fructose corn syrup and avoid it. Keep it out of your diet, and you will prevent many chronic health issues like diabetes, cancer, and other metabolic diseases. Since diabetes is more common in soft drink users, I often call soft drinks – "Diabetes in a bottle." The excess sugar and acidity actually create havoc in our cells.

Artificial sweeteners such as aspartame and sucralose are not better choices for sweeteners. The most common side effects of aspartame are headaches, increased joint pain, and worsening of premenstrual symptoms. Avoidance of all artificial sweeteners is recommended since they make us crave sugar in other forms. Recent research shows that aspartame also causes breakdown of the muscle. Artificial sweeteners trick your body into believing it is getting glucose in the cells. To make energy we need some glucose and our body will take it from our muscles when it needs it, making them weak. (Newman, 2018). Sucralose has research studies showing that it weakens the integrity of our intestinal lining causing "leaky gut syndrome." (Harpaz, 2016).

Avoid soft drinks to improve your health. The long-term effects of drinking carbonated beverages are not realized for some time. The longer you put these toxins in your system, the harder it will be to reverse the consequences. Many people report that when they stop drinking carbonated drinks, especially dark colas, they feel better overall.

Specific Remedies to Relieve Pain

Homeopathic Remedies

Homeopathy is a type of energy discipline that looks at particular symptoms of the fibromyalgia patient and matches them to a homeopathic remedy that fits the symptoms. There are classical homeopathic remedies that help with fibromyalgia pain very well and very quickly. Also, there are homeopathic combination remedies that support the metabolic imbalances found in fibromyalgia. I see more rapid relief using homeopathic remedies along with nutritional support than with just dietary changes.

As was shared earlier, homeopathic medicine philosophy believes that a person is not sick because he has an illness, but that he has an illness because he is sick and needs to heal. The illness is the symptom profile showing up, and the sickness is the metabolic imbalance causing the symptoms. It is critical to find the cause of the symptoms to actually promote healing. Homeopathic remedies provide the energy we need to sustain optimal health. Homeopathic combination remedies are often used to remind the body how to do what it already knows how to do but has forgotten due to stressful experiences.

Homeopathic medicine officially began in the early 1800s by Samuel Hahnemann. He was a medical doctor in Hungary that started the process of matching symptoms to the effects of natural substances. Homeopathy looks at each person's distinct symptoms and finds a remedy that matches the symptoms to improve the health of the whole system. Many of the principles of homeopathy are variations of conventional medicine principles. The "Law of Similars" is based on the principle of "like cures like." A small, diluted dose of a substance will stimulate the body to control its symptoms by healing and restoring balance. If the substances are consumed in large doses, they will cause the same type of symptoms the person is experiencing.

One example of the Law of Similars is using the remedy Apis for a sore throat or sunburn. The symptoms of a sore throat are burning, redness, swelling and stinging pain. The same symptoms occur with sunburn. Also, the same symptoms occur with a bee sting. The remedy Apis is made from a honey bee and is given to anyone displaying those similar symptoms. In vaccination and allergy therapy, a minimal amount of the bacteria or allergen is given to stimulate the tissues to create antibodies to these bacteria. Allergy shot therapy is similar to the "like cures like" principle.

The following remedies most often fit the symptoms of fibromyalgia and are chosen depending on the specific symptoms of the client. These are common remedies available in many health food stores. They come in small tubes containing tiny lactose sugar pellets that have the homeopathic remedy absorbed into the pellets. Three pellets are the recommended dosage, taken one to three times per day depending on the potency. The potencies in homeopathy are in Xs or C's. The 6X, 12X, or 30X, and the 6C, 12C, and 30C are common potencies found in health food stores. If the number is in the lower range, you will probably need to take the remedy more often to see results. With a 30X, or a 30C, potency, you may see results after just a few doses.

The most common remedy I recommend for muscle trauma and pain is **Arnica montana**. Arnica is an herb that can be applied topically as a cream on specific areas of bruising and pain. Arnica is often taken as a homeopathic remedy in pellet form internally, to work more deeply on the trauma that is affecting the muscles. Arnica improves circulation and reduces both emotional and physical trauma trapped in the muscles. Arnica is the best remedy after a traumatic event, like an accident that may have caused the onset of fibromyalgia. Try Arnica 30c pellets as your first choice for fibromyalgia muscle pain.

Rhus toxicodendron is another common homeopathic remedy for fibromyalgia pain. This remedy is made from the poison ivy plant. Rhus tox is best for stiffness that gets better once the client starts moving and when cold damp weather affects pain. Rhus toxicodendron is often used to relieve arthritis symptoms with pain in the joints due to ligament strains. The Rhus toxicodendron remedy helps with restlessness and anxiety about the pain. (Hershoff, 1996)

Bryonia is another homeopathic remedy that has opposite symptoms from the Rhus toxicodendron remedy. With Bryonia, the pain is worse on moving, so the slightest movement makes the pain worse. The client tends to be more irritable and doesn't like to be touched. Bryonia helps when there are pressure headaches, and the muscles feel hard. Another indication for Bryonia is when warmth makes the pain worse and cool applications feel better.

Magnesium phosphoricum is a homeopathic remedy to use when there are cramps and spasms with radiating pain. Neuralgic pains improve with warmth. Also, there is generalized muscle weakness especially in the arms and hands, and the fingertips may become stiff and numb. This remedy is made from magnesium phosphate and does similar actions as nutritional magnesium, yet in an energetic way.

Hypericum is a classical homeopathic remedy that helps heal nerve pain. Hypericum is helpful when there is numbness and tingling in the hands or feet, or radiating pain from one area to another. Hypericum can help with depression too, since it is an energetic version of the St. John's Wort plant.

Homeopathic remedies are also available in formulas of two or more substances mixed in combination. Formulas are a user-friendly way to use homeopathic remedies since the indications for their use are extremely clear. The practice of several substances combined in formulas provides a broad effect not available in a single remedy. One combination I recommend is Injurotox that has Arnica, Bryonia, Rhus tox, Magnesium phos, and Hypericum, in various potencies, plus many other synergetic ingredients that help heal traumas and injuries.

Single classical remedies work well when the specific symptoms are known, and when a higher potency of a remedy is desired but not available in a formula. Formula products usually contain potencies in the 3x, 6x, or 12x range. Two hundred years of homeopathic clinical experience proves that the higher the potency, the deeper and faster the remedy acts. When you have severe pain, you may see a more rapid benefit from the 30c potency. Use higher potency classical remedies when you are confident that they match your distinctive symptoms.

The use of lower potencies, such as the 6th or 12th potency, is indicated when general symptoms are used to find the remedy, or you can consider using a homeopathic formula. Lower potency combination remedies need to be taken more often to get a similar effect. At first, when there is the highest amount of pain and discomfort, the combination remedy may need to be taken every hour. Usually, after four doses, the frequency can be reduced to three times per day. If no improvement is noticed after a few days, it may not be the correct remedy, and other remedies should be considered.

In the releasing toxins section, I explained how other homeopathic remedy combinations are used to drain chemical toxins from the building up in the tissues. These drainage remedies are essential to consider when toxins are stuck in the tissues and are causing pain due to congestion. Many homeopathic remedy combinations work to help reduce pain on many levels.

Homeopathic remedies must be an integral part of a protocol to reduce fibromyalgia symptoms. I often recommend one classical remedy along with a combination formula that supports the overall cause of illness. The use of these remedies will reduce stress held in the muscle tissues, and will allow the pain to be relieved in a shorter period. The relief of pain that homeopathic remedies can provide will make it easier to create more lifestyle changes since you will feel better and have more energy more quickly.

Essential Oils

When you have fibromyalgia, you look for ways to reduce pain quickly. Essential oils work on fibromyalgia pain to alleviate aches, clear your brain fog, and increase energy. Essential oils along with homeopathic remedies are safe complementary therapies that can work along with any other therapies.

You can use these essential oils topically, in a hot bath, or a diffuser as aromatherapy. I like to combine peppermint, lavender, and cypress in a roller ball to use on specific points of pain. I use fractionated coconut oil to fill one-half of the roller ball and then fill the rest with equal amounts of these three essential oils.

Peppermint oil reduces pain, and the energizing scent can help clear brain fog and fatigue. Peppermint oil works as an antispasmodic to reduce muscle spasms or cramps. It also helps with sleep and improves circulation to reduce aches and pains. Peppermint oil is known for its benefits in reducing headaches. Peppermint oil may also improve memory, boost nervous system health, and reduce congestion.

Lavender oil can help reduce pain, improve mood, and helps with sleep issues. It is a potent analgesic oil, and even works with osteoarthritis. This essential oil is often in combinations for fibromyalgia symptoms.

Cypress oil works to increase circulation in the connective tissue. I always add it to a roller ball combination for pain. It can also reduce fatigue and stress.

Other essential oils that are often used to reduce fibromyalgia pain are:

Eucalyptus oil helps with muscle aches and soreness by improving blood circulation and flushing toxins from the tissues. It is known as a decongestant for the respiratory system because it helps reduce chronic inflammation.

Ginger oil helps with dizziness and nausea. Ginger is also known for blocking pain, reducing muscle spasms, and lowering inflammation by increasing antioxidant activity.

Helichrysum oil is often used for fibromyalgia pain, promising to relieve muscle pain and tension. It's an anti-inflammatory and has anti-oxidant properties that help reduce swelling and improves circulation.

CBD Oil For Fibromyalgia

Cannabis sativa made from hemp oil may also help reduce hypersensitivity to pain. Cannabidiol (CBD) oil is one of 100 chemical compounds found in cannabis sativa that is responsible for many of medical marijuana's health benefits without the perception altering side-effects.

CBD oil is different than medical marijuana that contains the psychoactive compound THC (delta-9-tetrahydrocannabinol.) CBD hemp oil with extremely low (less than 0.3 percent THC) is not part of the FDA Controlled Substance Act included in the Agriculture Improvement Act of 2018, making it a legal substance under federal law.

CBD oil may inhibit the nerve pathways that send pain signals between the brain and the body. Lack of neurotransmitters, including GABA, in the endocannabinoid system may be a cause of chronic pain. Taking CBD oil can increase these neurotransmitters helping to shift reactions to this cause of pain. (Russo, 2016)

From experience, many clients notice various results when using CBD oil for pain. Some see results quickly, and others do not see results at all. I recommend beginning slowly with a lower strength and increase the number of drops until results are seen. Common results are improvements in sleep, reduction of anxiety, and less hypersensitivity to pain. Use high quality CBD oil supplements that do not have filler oils found in many over-the-counter cheaper supplements.

CBD oil can be one of many supplements that reduce fibromyalgia symptoms. Experiment with a combination of homeopathic remedies, essential oils, CBD oil, and nutritional supplements to see what works to manage or eliminate your symptoms.

Bodywork, Energy Therapies, and Exercise for Pain Reduction

Treatment of fibromyalgia requires a comprehensive approach. The doctor, client and other health practitioners together play an active role in the management of fibromyalgia. Studies show that light movement exercises, such as swimming, tai chi, and walking, improve muscle fitness and reduce muscle pain and tenderness. Often heat applications and massage also give relief. Patients with fibromyalgia may benefit from a combination of light exercise, massage therapy, and relaxation.

Massage therapy can decrease fibromyalgia pain by relaxing muscles and improving circulation, which helps to get more oxygen to the muscles and remove toxins. Twenty-five percent of the participants in the research study used massage as a method to relieve pain. Most massage sessions are from one hour to one and one-half hours long. Other specific bodywork techniques are myofascial release and trigger point therapy. Myofascial release works deeply in the tissues to loosen up connective, or myofascial tissue and allow the muscles to relax and improve blood flow. Trigger point therapy involves holding specific pressure points to break up lymph stagnation and reduce tender point pain.

The fibromyalgia tender points develop in two ways. Local injury to tissues causes tearing in the fibers of muscles, tendons, ligaments, and the tissue lining the outside of the bone called the periosteum. These tears are also soft tissue injuries. Due to continuing stress, these tears do not heal. This persistent stress in the muscles near these tender points slows the flow of blood to the injured tissue and impairs the healing response. Typically, these points are not painful unless there is some injury to the localized area.

Acupuncture treatments can be very beneficial for reducing the pain of fibromyalgia without medications. Acupuncture uses a theory that meridians, or energy pathways, link the organs with the nervous system. By placing hair-thin needles in specific points along these meridians, circulation improves, and lymph flow more freely. Acupuncture also stimulates our body's painkillers, called endorphins. It also affects hormones and neurotransmitters that transmit nerve impulses so it can decrease hypersensitivity to pain.

PEMF Therapies

Another form of healing becoming more popular is Pulsed Electro-Magnetic Therapies (PEMF). There are a variety of devices used to improve circulation and voltage in the muscle tissues. Some devices can measure the voltage at specific points on the body. If the voltage is low, the underlying tissue does not have the energy to heal well. These devices add voltage to the cells to increase circulation and the healing ability, reducing pain very well. I use two different devices in my office depending on the needs of the client. Many clients get better energy and less anxiety overall, along with pain reduction.

I became interested in the Ondamed PEMF device because of its ability to help people with Lyme disease in just 12 to 15 sessions. This German-made device helps improve cellular energy for anxiety, pain, sleep, and even digestive imbalances. We give specific frequencies to the client depending on the results of individualized tests showing their need for nervous system energy balancing.

My newest device is the Tennant Biomodulator. The biomodulator is a portable hand-held device that will measure the voltage on the skin showing the energy in the underlying muscle tissue to heal. If the voltage is less than 20 mv, then there isn't enough energy to function well. Proper voltage is in the 25 to 30 mv area. When the voltage is over 40 mv, ideally in the 50 mv range, then healing is occurring. (Tennant,

2010). This device also helps improve the energy in the cell membrane. Cell membrane energy is essential to help nutrients get into the cells. I use this device on specific areas of pain, often knees, necks, backs, shoulders, and hands. There is a special attachment that I also use to energize all of the muscle battery packs in the whole body. For most people, they go from fatigued to energized in less than 10 minutes.

Relaxation

Finding time each day to relax the physical body and reduce mental overactivity helps to relieve built up stress. Just by taking a few minutes during the day to rest in a comfortable position with no background noise can have a similar effect to getting an hour-long nap. Listening to slow, meditative music can help to quiet the mind. At first, it may take some time to feel like your brain is willing to slow down, but with practice, you will be able to do it more quickly.

I also like to do a focused relaxation technique Dr. John Assaraf teaches in his NeuroGym program. This relaxation process helps you increase your awareness and become more self-confident. When you are feeling anxious, first take six deep breaths in through the nose and out through your mouth. While relaxed, become aware of your physical, mental and emotional state related to the activity that is stressing you now. Then ask yourself what intention do you want in this situation? Do you want to be frustrated? Or would you rather be calm and focused so you can respond better? Once you know what you want to experience, find one simple action to move you toward that intention. This focus exercise moves you out of a reactive state, and into a state where you have more control.

Exercise

Exercise helps everyone to stay healthy. Exercise has many benefits for the whole body. It moves stress out of the body and even helps with depression. Exercise helps to rejuvenate the cardiovascular system by strengthening the heart, lowering the heart rate and blood pressure, improving oxygen delivery into the cells and increasing blood supply to the muscle. Exercise helps mental function by relieving anxiety and tension, increases self-esteem and improves sleep patterns. Exercise enhances the muscle and joints by increasing muscle strength and flexibility, strengthening bones, and improving posture.

Before doing sustained exercise, including walking, stretching exercises help to reduce congestion in the muscles and get the muscles prepared for movement. Warm up with a few whole body motions to get the circulation flowing before beginning the stretching exercises. Stretching at the end of the workout or walk also helps to relax the muscles and move the acid out, so they do not get sore.

Even though we often think we get enough movement in our lives through daily activities such as housework, our exercise program needs to include an elevation in the heart rate for some time. Some examples of types of exercise that are helpful, but don't make the pain worse are walking, swimming, and exercise bicycles. Walking at a regular pace for 20 minutes 3 to 4 days per week can be extremely helpful to the system. Water exercise in warm water helps to relax the muscles without excess strain. Tai chi includes gentle movement exercises that increase circulation and flexibility without injury.

Simple movements often help to reduce the pain of fibromyalgia. Many of the participants in the study felt better with gentle exercise. Keep moving your body to help reduce stiffness and congestion. Finding a healthy exercise program that you can stick with is essential. I believe the best exercise program is the one that you enjoy and often do. I often recommend Dr. Zach Bush's "4 Minute Exercise" as a natural starting point. You can find it on a YouTube video showing how this exercise increases nitric oxide in your cells that indicate better circulation. (Bush, 2017)

Developing Your Program

So now what? You are probably asking - "What do I need to do to reduce MY pain?"

If you have read all the previous chapters, you have an understanding of what causes and helps relieve fibromyalgia pain. Do you have insight into what you need to do now? Or do you need to get more specific on identifying YOUR cause of suffering? Just by reading about concepts and ideas to create change, doesn't mean they are automatically put into motion. Now you get to decide what will work best for you and actually try it.

The following plan moves you through the 6 Root Causes of Symptoms elements: (Fisslinger, 2018). Take time to answer the following questions in a journal. Journaling helps to focus your energy in understanding your specific symptoms and triggers.

<u>Organ Tissue</u>

To get in touch with your pain it is important to ask these questions and identify location and perceptions you are having:

- o What organ tissue do you feel is most affected by your symptoms?
- o Are your nerves, striated muscle, fascia, adrenal, or thyroid stressed?

- Where exactly are your symptoms? Find the main location and identify the dominant side.
- What do you feel when you connect to the organ?
- Is the energy flowing or stuck?

You probably have overlapping organs affecting your pain response. Release the main area of organ tissue reaction that you feel with the following elements.

<u>Stress Triggers</u>

- What causes your pain to get worse?
- Is there a visual picture or recurring movie you see that creates pain?
- Is someone giving you the same verbal message all the time that triggers the pain?
- Is it your self-talk that is bringing you down?
- Is there a nagging feeling you have that is creating this recurring pain?
- Is there a conditioned reflux or habit pattern that triggers a stress reaction?
- How and when did your fibromyalgia symptoms begin?
- Did your symptoms start slowly?
- Or did they start after a traumatic event or change in your life?

The initiating event is a good clue of the underlying cause of your symptoms. For example, one client remembers her symptoms starting slowing while working with a manager she didn't like. Another client recognizes her symptoms beginning right after a car accident. So the first example would be emotional or mental stress creating her painful symptoms. The second example shows that physical trauma, probably with some emotional trauma, was the main acute cause. Discovering the initial stressful event and how you are continuing to react to this event now, will help you figure out the way to remove the root cause of the painful symptoms. When we don't fully process stressful events, we relive them in our daily lives until they are handled.

Emotions

Remember that emotions are energy in motion. Energy exists in all tissues of our body. We feel this energy as emotions. So when you have feelings, you are experiencing the movement of this energy. If we hide our feelings, we numb out our energy. It is necessary to feel this movement to help discharge it.

- o Which emotions do you feel in your organ tissue?
- o Are they trapped emotions, or could they be inherited emotions?
- o Is there a Chinese organ relationship of emotions affecting your flow of energy?
- o What action will you take to release or shift this emotion?

I like to use a 3 step process called "Feel, Want, Willing." Become aware of what you are feeling. Where is this sensation in your body? What do you intend to experience with this emotion? And then what action will you do to change the situation?

Get help to do emotional clearing techniques to remove layers of stress caused by trapped emotions. Find a positive emotion to focus on, and a simple action to remind you of this positive emotion in your daily life.

Beliefs

Beliefs are reinforced patterns in your brain coming from memories, personal experiences, and your perceptions of reality. Beliefs are the way we interpret the world and our understandings, and they color everything we say, think, and do. We become what we feel and what we do day after day. Habits eventually define us. Our brain creates habits to save us energy by generating familiar automatic tasks.

- Are there mental conflicts, or self-talk patterns, causing you stress?
- What are your consistent limiting beliefs?
- What is the ideal outcome you want?
- What can you learn from this experience to help you be in control?
- What can help you let go of this blocked energy?
- How do you want to react, feel, think, behave instead?
- What can you say to align your mind with your body?

Mental factors such as anxiety level and thought processes affect your health. Do you positively talk to yourself, or do you tend to put yourself down? What level of worry do you hold inside your organs daily? The amount of self-discipline, willingness, and determination you possess are factors that will significantly influence your ability in making lifestyle changes.

Understanding how true healing occurs, and being committed to incorporate changes to create healing, will enable the healing process to transpire. The patterns of our health come on from habits in our lives. Changing lifestyle, dietary, emotional, and mental habits will transform our healing ability. Generally, it takes one year of healing for every four years of living a toxic lifestyle, or one month for every four months. Everyone is different, so improvements are dependent on the strength of the whole body, including mental and emotional stability.

Social

Connections to family and friends are essential for balanced health. Environmental reactions affect our ability to respond to stress, and can affect our relationships, also.

- o Who do you depend on, and who depends on you?
- o Do you feel the love around you?
- o Do you allow love inside you?
- o How do you react to your environment?
- o Are you sensitive and react inappropriately to your environment?
- o How do toxins and microbes affect your health currently?
- o Have you considered where you can detox your environment?

Create positive social connections by uplifting others. Talk about common interests and be clear on your expectations with friends and family. Don't assume others know what you want. Relationship problems come when people anticipate others know what they expect. By enriching others with positive exchanges everyone will feel better.

Lifestyle

- o Are there daily habits you can improve?
- o Do you need help in your diet, sleep, or energy support?
- o Are you willing to take the time to test your pH and discover how your metabolism is functioning?
- o What type of remedies will support your needs during both the stress and regeneration phases well?
- o Did you complete the fibromyalgia pain quizzes?
- o Which area do you plan to focus on first?
- o What actions can you take to improve your most pain causing area?

Every day I see clients who take small specific actions and make significant improvements in their relief of fibromyalgia pain. Making habit changes often causes discomfort. We have to get out of our comfort zone to move forward. Challenges are good for physical, mental and emotional growth. Putting into practice even just a few of the many recommendations can make a big difference.

Energetic Testing to Improve Awareness

Remember, we have better health through awareness. Are there mental patterns, or sleep issues, from stress habits that are causing chronic pain? Stress is often a vague feeling that is difficult to explain and pinpoint the exact cause. That's one reason I do the Zyto Limbic Stress Assessment in my office to help clients understand what is causing their stress. We look at organs, food stressors, emotional reactions, nutritional imbalances, environmental toxins, immune reactions, and hormones. Limbic Stress Assessment involves communicating with the limbic system, part of the subconscious mind that controls autonomic responses.

The limbic system regulates our emotional behaviors and instinctual responses to our environment. We react to environmental toxins as perceived threats, and then make perceptions based on our past experiences. Then, we control our actions based on these new sensory preferences.

An out-of-balance limbic system will create distorted threat reactions. As we continually seek to protect ourselves, we will acquire symptoms to defend us from even low levels of toxins. We will react excessively to odors and noises creating headaches, fatigue, and dizziness. Threat messages will get priority, and lead to uncontrollable reactions that are not appropriate to the aggravation. The body is put on high alert, adrenaline pumps through the muscles, senses are heightened, and we either fight, flight or freeze. Our feelings reach the cortex of the brain and thought patterns become habitual and permanently program your body to stay in survival mode.

Understanding what you are reacting to, and calming the limbic stress related to that reaction, helps simplify your healing process. Use energy clearing techniques and homeopathic remedies to desensitize you to these excessive reactions of your limbic system. Lifestyle Prescription Health Coaches have a specific technique to help rebalance your limbic system. Limbic system clearing happens by finding the root cause and unblocking layers of stress triggers in a set of coaching sessions.

Remember that health promotion is more than prevention of disease. Being healthy involves taking responsibility for your health, your choices. Don't live with bad habits and expect a doctor or medication to counteract your lifestyle and symptoms. Being aware of your health is the first step to healing. Here are five steps to change habits and create real-life solutions.

Steps to Change Habits and Create Real Life Solutions

1. Know the cause of your symptoms and be clear about what you want to improve. You have the results from your fibromyalgia pain quizzes showing your most out-of-balance area. What do you want to change? Is it being tired of chronic pain or fatigue? Why do you need this? Is it to be able to do something or be someone different? Knowing the cause of your symptoms helps create motivation to change. Having a goal and being clear on your reason to change is necessary.

2. Pick one area and improve it. Focus on making small habit changes one at a time. You read some recommendations that you know you can do. Make one simple change at a time.

Do one adjustment for a week or more, and then add a new action, gradually multiplying your success.

3. Let go of social stressors. Are there people who expect you to act a certain way? You are a unique individual. Be authentic! Stay in your integrity, live by your values. Integrity reduces social stressors when you do what you know is right for you. You may have expectations that may be holding you back, too. Find them and shift them. Is there any activity you are doing now that takes your energy away from you? Adjust your activities to fit your new lifestyle. Check your environment. We have places that trigger our habits. Do you see patterns for your symptoms depending on where you are, or what you are doing?

4. Calibrate and adjust your daily actions to fit new behaviors. We are all creatures of habit, and to change we have to shift triggers that moved us toward old habits. When creating new solutions, consistently watch your results and adjust to keep moving forward. Automate or systemize your actions so that by consistently repeating your new behaviors they get programmed in your limbic system.

5. Increase love and support in your life. Social connections in your life help keep moving you forward. Desiring trusted associates is one reason many successful people have a coach. Professional athletes have coaches that watch their actions and tell them how to improve. Health coaches listen and help you discover what you are saying or what you are doing that is affecting your health, and then keep you motivated toward new actions. Find a coach to give you positive attention. Coaches often remind you to reward yourself after accomplishing goals.

As a Lifestyle Prescriptions® Health Coach, I often challenge clients to change habits creating symptoms. A common challenge is a dietary change. For example, if you want to see how your diet affects your pain level, do this: Go on a no sugar and no processed grains, like flour, diet for 21 days. Sugar creates stickiness in your cell lining, causing inflammation and hardening of the artery wall. Have you ever dripped maple syrup on a table? Remember how sticky it gets? That toughening in the tissues lowers circulation that leads to stiffness and pain. Grains turn to glucose too, so the lower amount of processed grains you eat, often the better you feel.

Look at your plate when you eat. Do you know it should be 50% fruit and vegetables at each meal? Fruit and vegetable provide extra fiber. Fiber slows the processing of sugar for energy. Even though fruits have sugar, they are allowed on the no sugar program, because of the fiber in them. Mainly fruits and vegetables, and minimal sugars and processed grains are common recommendations for positive dietary changes.

As creatures of habit, dietary changes are often the easiest physical challenges to try. How long can you go before you fall back to your previous beliefs and actions about food choices? We don't have to eat perfectly all the time. Challenging yourself in this area helps build up your awareness for transformation and strengthens your determination.

Many factors cause fibromyalgia symptoms. Systemic imbalances create pain in all areas of the body. Systemic imbalances also generate other symptoms commonly found associated with fibromyalgia including chronic fatigue, anxiety, depression, and weak immune system function. Only by improving the overall health through the use of a combination of therapeutic techniques can the symptoms be indeed reduced or relieved. Choose the supplements, homeopathic remedies, and essential oils that support your regeneration phase, and reduce reenacting the stress phase.

A whole lifestyle program is necessary for relieving fibromyalgia. Adequate amounts of sleep are required so that the body can regenerate during the night. Daily stretching exercises will help to keep circulation flowing through the muscles. Learning to meditate and relax the mind will help balance stress factors.

Diet, of course, is critical. Eating whole natural foods will gradually improve your energy level. Consume many dark green vegetables in the diet, and use whole food supplements for the antioxidants and absorbable calcium they contain. Include supplements with magnesium and malic acid, along with the B-complex vitamins to reduce stress and improve circulation in the muscles. Adding essential fatty acids helps improve the absorption of nutrients into the cells by increasing cell flexibility and improving cell function.

Look at your specific symptoms, and see where you may have nutritional and metabolic weaknesses. Then select the supplements and dietary changes that will benefit you the most. Take small action steps and pay attention to the changes you see. Redo the fibromyalgia pain quizzes monthly and see what improvements you see. Fibromyalgia symptoms can absolutely be reversed and managed when improvements are made to recover healthy functioning of the whole body by supporting the inherent healing ability.

It is so important to take into account all six root causes of symptoms. We cannot make long-term changes if we have stuck social/mental/emotional patterns that hold us back from true healing. Many factors will influence the length of time it will take for you to reverse your fibromyalgia symptoms. By learning how to use all aspects of this program in your daily lifestyle, you will have the best likelihood to create the health you desire.

Works Cited

Abraham, G. F. (1992;3). Management of Fibromyalgia: Rational for the Use of Magnesium and Malic Acid. *Journal of Nutritional Medicine*, 49-59.

ACR. *Fibromyalgia Tender Points*. American College of Rheumatology.

Beinfield, H. K. (1992). *Between Heaven and Earth: A Guide to Chinese Medicine*. Ballantine Books.

Burrascano, J. (2017). *Lyme Disease Symptons and Signs*. Lyme Disease Association.

Bush, Z. (2017, September 5). *4 Minute Workout*. Retrieved from YouTube: https://www.youtube.com/watch?v=PwJCJToQmps &list=PLGLEnbPwqwqeF5ueyhKdG_rEQPxXYqn70

Campbell, S. e. (1983; 26). Clinical Characteristics of Fibrositis, A Blinded Controlled Study of Symptoms and Tender Points. *Arthritis Rhem*, 817-824.

Choy, E. (2015). The Role of Sleep in Pain and Fibromyalgia. *National Review of Rheumatology*, 513-520.

DeMartini, J. (2013). *The Values Factor*. NY, NY: Berkley Publishing Group.

Draper, H. (1984). Urinary Malondialdehyde as an Indicator of Lipid Peroxidation in the Diet and in the Tissues. *Lipids*, 836-843.

EPA. (2010). *Chemicals in Food*. Retrieved from Environmental Protection Agency: http://www.epa.gov/ogwow/ccl/cclfs.html

EWG. (2015, October 1). *Organic Diet Reduced Children's Exposure to Pesticide.* Retrieved from Enviromental Working Group: https://www.ewg.org/enviroblog/2015/10/organic-diet-reduced-children-s-exposure-pesticides

Fisslinger, J. R. (2018). *The 6 Root Causes of All Symptoms.* www.Lifestyle Prescriptions.TV.

Harpaz, D. L. (2016). Measuring Artificial Sweetener Toxicity Using a Bioluminescence Bacterial Panel. *Molecules,* p. 2454.

Hershoff, A. (1996). Homeopathy for Musculoskeletal Healing. North Atlantic Books.

Jones, G. A. (2014, October 16). *American College of Rheumatology.* Retrieved from Prevalance of Fibromyalgia and Modified 2010 Classification Criteria: https://doi.org/10.1002/art.38905

LifestylePrescriptions®.TV. (2018). *Sefl-Healing Made Easy.* Retrieved from Lifestyle Prescriptions®: www.lifestyleprescriptions.tv

Meeker, J. (2012). Exposure to Environmental Endocrine Disruptors and Child Development. *Archives of Pediatric Adolescence Medicine, 32.*

Nelson, B. (2007). *The Emotion Code.* Wellness Unmasked Publishing.

Newman, T. (2018, April 23). Artificial Sweeteners May Damage Blood Vessels. *Medical News Today.*

NFA. (n.d.). *10 Things FM Patients Need to Know.* Retrieved from www.FMAware.org

NFCPA. (n.d.). *FM Fact Sheet.* Retrieved from FMCP Aware: https://www.fmcpaware.org/fibromyalgia/fm-fact-sheet.html

Ortner, N. (2013). *The Tapping Solution.* Retrieved from 2013 Tapping World Summit: https://www.thetappingsolution.com/what-is-eft-tapping/

Robbins, T. (2017). *Tony Robbins.* Retrieved January 26, 2019, from Do You Need to Feel Significant: https://www.tonyrobbins.com/mind-meaning/do-you-need-to-feel-significant/

Russo, E. (2016, July 28). Clinical Endocannabinoid Deficiency Reconsidered: Current Research Support the Theory in

Migraine, Fibromyalgia, Irritable Bowel, and Other Treatment Resistant Syndromes. *Cannabinoid Research*, pp. Vol 1, No. 1.

Tennant, J. (2010). *Healing is Voltage The Handbook 3rd Edition.* Independent Publishing.

Wilke, W. (1996L 100(1)). Fibromyalgia: Recognizing and addressing the multiple interrrlated factors. *Postgraduate Medicine*, 153-170.

Wilson, J. (2001). *Adrenal Fatigue.* Smart Publications.

Wolf, F. (1986). The Clinical Syndrome of Fibrositis. *American Journal of Medicine*, 7-13.

Wolfe, M. F. (1990, February). *1990 criteria for Classification for Fibromyalgia.* Retrieved from American College of Rheumatology: https://doi.org/10.1002/art.170330203

Zareba, G. (2008, Dec). New Treatment Options in the Management of Fibromyalgia: role of pregabalin. *Neuropsychiatric Disease Treatment*, 1193-1201.

Index

CPSIA information can be obtained
at www.ICGtesting.com
Printed in the USA
BVHW030146060822
643962BV00009B/501